D0894194

New Pathways to Medical Education

New Pathways to Medical Education

Learning to Learn at Harvard Medical School

EDITED BY DANIEL C. TOSTESON,
S. JAMES ADELSTEIN, AND SUSAN T. CARVER

Harvard University Press
Cambridge, Massachusetts
London, England
1994

Printed in the United States of America

This book is printed on acid-free paper.

LIBRARY OF CONGRESS CATALOGING-IN-PUBLICATION DATA

New pathways to medical education : learning to learn at Harvard Medical School / edited by Daniel C. Tosteson, S. James Adelstein, and Susan T. Carver.
p. cm.
Includes bibliographical references and index.
ISBN 0-674-61738-X (alk. paper) (cloth)
ISBN 0-674-61739-8 (paper)
1. Harvard Medical School. 2. Medicine—Study and teaching—Massachusetts—Boston. 3. Curriculum change. I. Tosteson, D. C., 1925– . II. Adelstein, S. J. III. Carver, Susan T.
[DNLM: 1. Harvard Medical School. 2. Curriculum. 3. Education, Medical. W 18 N555 1994]
R747.H28N48 1994
610'.71'174461—dc20
DNLM/DLC
for Library of Congress

94-11196
CIP

Contents

Foreword

August G. Swanson

Until 1987, the education of medical students in North America had been largely unchanged since the beginning of the twentieth century, when the curricular pattern introduced at Johns Hopkins University, Harvard University, and the University of Michigan was adopted by 90 percent of medical schools in the United States and Canada: two years of courses in the basic sciences, followed by clinical clerkships. In curriculums following this paradigm, during the first two years students learn about the sciences basic to medicine by sitting through lectures in large groups, and demonstrate acquired basic science knowledge by taking multiple-choice examinations.

Many students view these first two years as barriers to their becoming doctors rather than as a period devoted to acquiring knowledge and learning skills that they will apply throughout their careers. Faculty members believe that students must gain clinical skills, but few faculty consider students' attainment of learning skills either important or a faculty responsibility.

Many have said that changing a curriculum is more difficult than moving a graveyard. Perhaps that is why there has been so little educational innovation by medical schools. Indeed, at most medical schools, medical student education has been the faculty's lowest priority. The Association of American Medical Colleges' 1984 report on the general professional education of physicians stated that "Despite frequent assertions that the general professional education of medical students is the basic mission of medical schools, it often occupies last place in the competition for faculty time and attention; graduate students, residents, research and patient care are accorded higher priorities." This book details how Harvard Medical School overcame the prevailing educational inertia and developed a curriculum and educational program consistent with preparing students to practice medicine in the twenty-first century. The New Pathway emphasizes both acquiring current knowledge and developing learning skills that will be used throughout physicians' professional lives.

Each medical school faculty has special talents and exists in a unique environment. The educational program developed at one school cannot simply be adopted wholesale by another. However, educational strategies that have demonstrated success in one school can be adopted by other institutions. This book details both these strategies and the planning and implementation of Harvard's New Pathway. It is offered as a stimulus and guide to other medical schools seeking effective ways to educate students who will practice in the twenty-first century.

New Pathways to Medical Education

1

Toward a New Medicine

Daniel C. Tosteson

In 1982, faculty, administrators, and students at Harvard Medical School developed and launched the program known as the New Pathway in General Medical Education, a sustained search by members of the faculty and their students for better methods of preparing for the practice of medicine and medical science. The following chapters, written by a number of the leaders involved in this initiative, describe different parts of the program. Here, however, in this introductory chapter, I want to explain why I consider this project to be essential, not only for the future of the Harvard Medical School but also for that of other academic medical centers, for the medical profession, and, most important, for the health of the people whom it serves.

The medicine of the twenty-first century will be very different from the medicine of today. The encounter between doctor and patient will be, as it has always been, a collaboration between two persons directed toward improving the health of the patient. But the scientific, technological, economic, and ethical conditions of medical practice are changing rapidly and will continue to do so. The task of medical education is to help people entering medicine to prepare to meet their professional obligations in this new context. The nature of the educational task must change as the nature of the profession changes. Harvard's New Pathway was created to explore the changing nature of general medical education.

The most powerful forces transforming medicine are the new

concepts of human health and disease created by recent discoveries in the natural sciences. We now recognize all living organisms to be open molecular systems operating in or near the steady state, constantly taking in and putting out matter and energy. From a physical point of view, these systems express the play of electromagnetism. Strong and weak nuclear forces, together with gravitation, set the conditions, but electromagnetic energy arriving on earth from the sun drives the chemical reactions that are the signature of life. It is this force that forms the bonds between atoms, permitting the formation of the molecules that comprise living systems.

In 1982, at a symposium commemorating the bicentennial of Harvard Medical School, Arthur Kornberg delivered a lecture titled "Understanding Life as Chemistry."[1] In it he argued forcefully for a concerted effort by the biomedical scientific community to isolate, identify, and characterize the molecules that constitute the human and other organisms. The current international effort to map and sequence the human genome can be viewed as one response to his plea. By September 1990, 1,820 of the approximately 10^5 coding human genes had been mapped.[2] Although this number represents only about 2 percent of the total, it also marks extraordinary progress, given that no human genes had been sequenced in 1975. Furthermore, no conceptual or technical barriers now stand in the way of completing the task; it is only a matter of how much time will be required. As this information becomes available, it will completely alter the conceptual framework within which physicians think and work.

One of the consequences of sequencing the human genome will be an increasing awareness of the connections between all living things: the homology of vitally important, and therefore highly conserved, genes between humans and other living forms as primitive as yeast indicates that we share a common ancestor with these microorganisms, which have been in existence for hundreds of millions of years. Another consequence will be increased attention to the exquisite complexity of the arrays of molecules that regulate metabolism. We will understand more and more that the balance of health and disease in the human population is an expression of biological evolution in action. We will know the variety of genetically related proteins produced by the natural selection of mutants. We will learn how the interindividual differences in number and kind of genetically determined macromolecules render each person more or less susceptible to potentially pathogenic conditions in the environment. We will become progressively more competent at matching genetic predisposition to environment in order to maximize health. These adjustments will be made not only by modifying external influences (for example, through control of diet) but also by altering gene expression (both through drugs that activate or repress the process and through the insertion of genes). Such are the rudiments of a contemporary vision of life as chemistry.

The proteins coded by genes and all the other molecules that make up the human body are manufactured in cells. The adult human organism is the result of between forty and fifty generations of cells arising from the fertilized ovum. Guided by its genomic blueprint and stimuli arising in its local environment, each of these approximately 10^{14} cells synthesizes the chemical parts of which it is made. Each of these parts must not only meet stringent molecular tolerances but also be positioned in the appropriate location in the cell. These locations are often in or on membranes surrounding the entire cell or organelles such as nuclei, mitochondria, and endoplasmic reticulum. This intracellular, macromolecular economy is also directed by gene products. Some of the cells formed during development—for example, neurons and spermatogonia—persist without further division as long as the organism lives. Others terminate by mechanisms other than division, such as ingestion by phagocytes (as with blood cells), loss to the environment (as with skin and epithelia of the gut), or programmed cell death. Such lost or destroyed cells are replaced by continuing division of appropriate stem cells. The science of cell biology seeks to reveal the mechanisms used by all cells to self-assemble, differentiate, function, and divide—to portray life as cells.

Many aspects of function, however, are more easily understood in terms of families of cells arranged in tissues and organs rather than in terms of individual cells. The custom of organizing the specialties of clinical medicine by organ systems is not only a result of the technological limitations of nineteenth- and twentieth-century medical science, but also a valid reflection of the fact that functions such as circulation, respiration, digestion, sensation, and movement of the human body are carried out by families of many specialized cells arranged in specific geometries. The rise of molecular and cell biology has added extraordinary texture to human physiology. We are slowly groping toward ways of thinking about the function of the entire organism enlightened by the realization that the action is taking place in cells, small volumes (approximately 10^{-12} to 10^{-13} liters) of dilute seawater, each containing an array of genetically determined macromolecules organized into various organelles and surrounded by thin (less than 10^{-6} centimeters) phospholipid and protein membranes.

Nowhere is the search for a new paradigm for biomedical science more evident than in human pharmacology. Drugs intended to modify functions such as gastric secretion[3] and regulation of blood pressure[4] are identified and/or designed as inhibitors of specific enzymes. Whether a specific inhibitor will modify function in the living organism is problematic until trials in animals and man have been conducted. The use of transgenic organisms to elucidate the function of genes may be viewed as a modern application of organismic physiology and pathology. The construction of a sophisticated physiology and pharmacology that incorporates the molecular and cellular texture will be an agenda for biologists and physicians for decades to come.

These momentous developments in the natural sciences are not alone in changing the conceptual basis of medicine. Discoveries in the social sciences also are yielding new perspectives. Human beings live in social groups. Most of what distinguishes us from our forebears is the result of cooperation between individual human beings organized into societies. We help one another, but we also make one another sick. Much of morbidity is determined by differences in the socioeconomic conditions in which people live. Medical anthropologists are identifying patterns of incidence and manifestations of disease in different populations.[5] These differences often can be correlated with social customs such as smoking, alcohol or other drug use, diet, waste disposal, and sanitation. Many of these factors are as evident in the United States as they are in so-called underdeveloped countries. Historians of medicine have laid bare the social correlates of different styles of medical practice in different human societies in successive historical periods.[6] Social scientists are making physicians much more aware of social determinants of morbidity as well as methods of practice.

The unprecedented growth in the sciences basic to medicine has spawned ever more potent technologies that are useful in medical practice and in medical science. Science and technology are symbiotic. New ways of observing our surroundings made possible by new devices such as electron microscopes, spectrometers for detecting electromagnetic radiation of various frequencies from X-rays to infrared, magnetic resonance detectors, mass spectrometers, chromatographic techniques for rapid separation of molecules by mass and charge—all have allowed the framing of questions that could not have been conceived previously and have permitted a more rigorous and stringent test of old hypotheses. Particularly noteworthy is the emergence of computers and related devices for managing information. Without all these technologies, projects like the mapping and sequencing of the human genome and the determination of the three-dimensional structure of proteins and other macromolecules would not be possible. The autocatalytic growth of science and technology seems likely to continue indefinitely.

The new technologies have transformed not only the methods of medical science but also the techniques of clinical practice. Modern physicians use an array of new diagnostic, preventive, and therapeutic tools. The extraordinary progress in noninvasive imaging, particularly by nuclear magnetic resonance, makes possible the detection of lesions that could not have been identified even a few years ago. Nuclear magnetic resonance will someday allow the noninvasive, on-line assay of chemical substituents of specific tissues.[7] Determination of the three-dimensional structure of the active sites of enzymes is opening the possibility of rational design of inhibitors that are candidates for effective drugs. Recombinant-DNA technology allows the production in microorganisms of any desired human protein, including growth hormone, insulin, and tissue plasminogen activator. In September 1990 the first clinical trial of gene therapy of an inherited human disease, adenosine deaminase deficiency, began. It will be followed by many more such interventions. A more sophisticated understanding of the immune system is allowing more degrees of freedom in transplantation of tissues and organs.

Demand for the design, production, and distribution of medical technologies has created a new growth industry that operates in parallel with the medical profession and without which modern medical practice would be impossible. This industry provides physicians with drugs, devices, and physical settings for the care of patients. The relation between the medical industry and the medical profession is becoming increasingly complex. Many physicians now play essential roles in the medical industry. Those who are also directly involved in the care of patients must always be clear that their primary commitment is to their patients rather than to the companies that provide them with necessary tools and workplaces. Likewise, medical scientists discovering the secrets of human biology must reach out to companies that will develop their discoveries into products useful to patients but not lose sight of their primary obligation to search for deeper insights. These interfaces between scholars and physicians on the one hand and the medical industry on the other must remain permeable but selective.

The increasing technical power of medicine has enlarged enormously the available range of feasible preventive and therapeutic interventions. The advent of coronary bypass surgery for patients at risk for myocardial infarction is a clear example. Each new technique for diagnosis and treatment has spawned a new pool of experts. Every specialty of medicine is differentiating into subspecialties; for example, ophthalmologists have subdivided into experts on the cornea, the retina, glaucoma, and so on. For reasons of conceptual appeal, compensation, and a lifestyle that allows for more balance among professional, family, and recreational activities, a larger and larger proportion of young doctors are choosing to enter these subspecialties. One consequence of this subspecialization is an undersupply of physicians providing primary care. Another result is the tendency toward providing comprehensive care through groups of subspecialists practicing together. Preserving attention to the personal needs of individual patients in these more complex clinical and technical settings is an enormous challenge to the profession.

Changes in the economics of medical care are also reshaping the medicine of the twenty-first century. The fee-for-service system persists in the United States, but it does so for the most part in conjunction with public and private third parties that provide patients with insurance to cover their expenses for medical care. Over 60 percent of Americans now have some form of health insurance. It has become commonplace for employers to purchase such insurance for their employees. Physicians increasingly negotiate for payment of their fees not with their patients but with one or more of these third parties. Frequently these negotiations deal not only with financial matters but also with the quantity and quality of the medical services rendered. The tone of these negotiations is partly captured by the new jargon; patients and their third-party representatives have become consumers, while physicians and other health professionals have become providers of medical care.

The superinflationary increase in the costs of medical care is another important economic sequela of the large increase in the range and power of technical interventions that doctors can make to alter the course of disease. During 1990 alone, expenses for health insurance paid by corporations for their employees rose by 21.6 percent.[8] Expressions of dissatisfaction about the apparently inexorable growth of medical costs have been increasingly loud and frequent. Corporations are demanding contracts from insurers and providers that constrain costs. These often involve agreements with health maintenance organizations (HMOs) or with groups of independent physicians.[9] These managed-care agreements generally assure patients a package of benefits for a predetermined price. They raise potential conflicts between the obligations of physicians to their patients and to their employers or payers. For medical reasons, the patient may require additional services, but the associated expense may be unacceptable to the payer. This is but one of the many ethical issues that will be faced by the physicians of the twenty-first century.

The most serious problem facing the medical system in the United States is not, however, escalating costs, but rather providing care for the 33 percent of the population who are now uninsured or inadequately insured. In 1965, with the passage of legislation mandating the Medicare and Medicaid programs, the nation started toward a medical care system that could be used by all citizens, independently of their capacity to pay. By 1980 the cost to the taxpayers had risen to a point where many voters and politicians began to question the feasibility of this goal. Since that time, efforts to constrain the costs and, thus, the benefits provided by these programs have intensified. Public general and mental hospitals have shrunk or closed. The impact on the availability of medical care to the poor and elderly has been disastrous. Advocates for reform of this situation remain relatively powerless. Physicians of the twenty-first century will not be able to avoid this massive problem.

At root, this problem is not primarily economic, but ethical. It is but one of many ethical issues with which physicians must deal. The increasing power of molecular medicine makes possible clinical interventions that a few years ago were only theoretical. Transplantation of organs began with kidneys of identical twins in 1953[10] but has now extended to permit transfer between unrelated individuals of not only kidney but also heart, liver, pancreas, and bone marrow. Advances in surgery of the fetus and newborn, as well as the capacity to diagnose genetic defects *in utero,* have opened the way to major corrections of errors of development during very early life. At the other end of the spectrum, physicians now have the capacity to sustain life indefinitely in individuals who cannot move or sense their surroundings. The personal and social consequences of these developments pose questions that cannot be answered by physicians alone, but require the participation of patients, families, lawyers, clergy, and others. On the other hand, doctors must participate fully in the development and implementation of ethical policies that will assure that the clinical uses of the new medicine accrue to the benefit of patients.

All these interconnected forces are transforming the medical profession and its related industries at an accelerating rate. What do these transformations portend for the future of medical education? Harvard Medical School's New Pathway explores these questions at both conceptual and organizational levels.

Conceptual issues include both content and process, substance and form. For example: What are the attitudes, skills, and knowledge that all medical students should share, irrespective of their ultimate professional career focus? What is the most cost-effective way in which faculties of medical schools and universities can help students to develop these qualities? These complex questions often generate strongly conflicting opinions among scholars. Nevertheless, there is growing agreement about the desirable directions for change in the content and process of general medical education.[11]

First, there is emerging consensus that attitudes and skills in learning and practicing are as important as or more important than the acquisition of technical knowledge during the course of general medical education. The incredible growth of knowledge in the sciences basic to medicine makes it literally impossible for students to acquire during medical school and to retain thereafter all the information necessary for a lifetime of effective practice. Rather, both as students and during their careers, physicians must nurture a commitment to learn whatever is pertinent to the health of their patients and develop the skills to learn whatever is necessary. Explicit attention to the cultivation of attitudes and skills, at the marginal expense of didactic exposure to information, is one of the axioms of the New Pathway project. The prime criterion for including a particular course or exercise in the curriculum is whether or not it will promote a permanent personal commitment to learning and help students to acquire a learning skill of lasting value.

The New Pathway does not, in the words of the great French physiologist Claude Bernard, "raise ignorance to a principle."[12] Rather, it views the construction of a framework of knowledge, ways of thinking about human beings in health and disease, as an essential component of an effective program of general medical education. The most important feature of such a framework is that it include *all* the determinants of health. It should express the Aristotelian aphorism that "medicine begins in philosophy, and philosophy ends in medicine." Such a philosophical framework for medicine should include at least three dimensions. First, it should recognize human beings as living organisms both closely related chemically and physically to all living organisms and also remarkably diverse, as revealed by modern molecular and cell biology.

Second, the framework of knowledge should view humans as members of society. Interactions between people have created all that distinguishes modern from primitive humans, including our capacity to practice medicine more effectively. All these developments flow from the ability of people to communicate reliably and to act cooperatively. These characteristics are the basis of learning. They allow us to know and to do more together than we can individually. Herbert Simon uses the term "docility" to describe these aspects of human behavior and argues that there are circumstances in which they may be selected for in evolution.[13] But humans' proclivity to live in close-knit groups also has pathological consequences. Proximity increases the chances of transmission of infectious diseases between individuals, and the emotions generated in relationships between people are often components in the etiology of psychopathology.

Third, physicians must view their patients not only as living organisms and members of society but also as unique individuals. This third dimension of the framework of knowledge that all physicians share is elaborated in the humanities, in history, literature, and the arts. Each clinical encounter is unique in time, place, and the participants involved. In the last analysis, the experience of illness and suffering is lonely. The physician is obliged to seek to reach through the boundary that separates the inside from the outside of the patient in order to understand and share the burden. The effectiveness of this transaction between persons is often crucial for accurate diagnosis and for compliance with plans for prevention or treatment.

If the promotion of attitudes and skills for continuing learning and the creation of an inclusive framework for medical knowledge are the appropriate content for general medical education, what are the best methods for cultivating such growth? The two essential components of the New Pathway methodology are student and problem. The entire program is designed to encourage students to assume personal responsibility for their learning. As much as possible, students are given the opportunity to choose how, where, when, and, to a significant extent, what to learn. Such choices are often the first and hardest steps toward learning outside the institutional setting. Furthermore, the program emphasizes learning in the context of real problems rather than along the lines of organized bodies of knowledge. The courses are generally interdepartmental and interdisciplinary.

A particular goal of this student-centered, problem-based approach is to develop physicians who practice "science in action" rather than attempting to apply learned formulas to clinical situations.[14] The aim is to build an awareness that the methods and insights of the natural and social sciences and the humanities basic to medicine are inseparable from the day-to-day practice of all kinds of medicine. To this end, from their first day students face clinical problems in the process of learning basic science, and they continue to confront scientific issues in clerkships toward the end of the sequence.

Computers and other information-managing devices are learning tools that all physicians will continue to use increasingly. Many students now enter medical school with some experience in using these devices. Most clinical settings already make heavy use of this technology in managing patient records. However, the capabilities of the hardware generally exceed the sophistication of the software available for learning and practicing medicine. The New Pathway promotes student and faculty involvement in creating new approaches to the use of computers in medical education.

Since the essence of the medical encounter is the interaction between two persons, a physician and a patient, the New Pathway provides experiences designed to encourage the development of the interpersonal skills necessary to understand and use this relationship for the benefit of the patient. Much of this effort occurs during a three-year sequence of tutorial sessions called Patient–Doctor that explores many aspects of this relationship, including the development of clinical skills such as physical diagnosis and history-taking through a consideration of issues in medical economics and ethics. In the third year it provides students with an opportunity to analyze and reflect on some of their clerkship experiences. The Patient–Doctor sequence is an enduring influence throughout the New Pathway curriculum.

The future direction of the program of general medical education at Harvard Medical School depends on organizational as well as conceptual reform. The difficult problems of choosing the most appropriate content and methods of education will be solved effectively only if faculty members dedicate adequate time and energy to the task. Before the initiation of the New Pathway project, the faculty of medicine at Harvard (and at many other research-intensive medical schools) devoted less than 5 percent of their effort to educating medical students. Moreover, their contributions were usually in the form of didactic expositions about their subspecialty of basic science or clinical medicine. Few were aware of the overall strategy of the educational program, and as a result curriculums were fragmented and uncoordinated. Students and faculty rarely had the opportunity to become personally acquainted. Student frustration, particularly with the first two years devoted to the basic sciences, was high.

To address these problems, the New Pathway organized faculty into units, called academic societies, to improve the coherence and coordination of the entire curriculum and to strengthen the personal relationships between students and faculty that underlie the growth of commitment to learning. The academic societies are envisioned as the organizations responsible for planning and implementing Harvard's program of general medical education by devising the comprehensive strategy and the specific tactics of the entire sequence of experiences that will enable students to move productively from the initial choice of medicine as a career to the point of entry into post-M.D. degree training. Currently this sequence of experiences occurs in at least three different sets of institutions: the colleges, the medical schools, and the teaching hospitals. No single group of faculty oversees the entire sequence. Moreover, even within the medical school, integration of the process is weak. The academic societies will devote most of their attention to this central segment, but they will also address the interfaces with the college and teaching hospital segments.

Another essential component of the New Pathway at Harvard Medical School is a group of educational professionals who have worked closely with the faculty, helping them to plan and implement the various courses, to improve their expository skills, and also to become effective tutors in small-group, problem-based sessions, where they serve less as sources of information and more as facilitators to help students acquire the attitudes and skills for independent learning. The educators and their staffs have also been essential for the development of the cases used in these tutorial sessions, assuming responsibility for each required course.

In the following pages we present information about the history, concept, and organization of the New Pathway project in the hope our experiences will stimulate physicians, medical scientists, and educators elsewhere to think more deeply and act more decisively to reform medical education. Such labors could benefit not only the medical profession but society in general. How to live productively and peacefully in an information-intensive social environment is a problem not limited to medicine. Despite spectacular progress in the development of computers and other information-management technologies, it seems likely that the accumulation of information will continue to outstrip the capacity of individual human beings to assimilate new data. Subspecialization will proceed ever more rapidly, and experts in different fields will become more and more isolated from one another. Nurturing the bonds that unite rather than divide professionals and scholars will become more difficult. Doing so will require fundamental changes in the way that we think about education. Recognition that learning and living are inseparable must become more a part of everyday life. The social roles of universities and professional schools will be more clearly directed toward preparing students for lives of learning. Educators in medicine can make a significant contribution toward this re-examination of higher education of all kinds.

However medical educators tackle reform, they are likely to encounter the same two issues that preoccupied the participants in the New Pathway project at Harvard Medical School. They will need to define and articulate a vision, a concept of the curriculum that includes both its content and its methods. Equally important, they must identify faculty organizations that will have the authority and responsibility for planning and implementing the program and for sustaining curricular innovation. Different institutions will select different paths appropriate to their particular circumstances. Ideally, each institution will share its experiences so that the entire academic medical community will gradually improve the quality of its programs of general medical education. The goal of medical education is to increase the ability of physicians to bring the practical benefits of the new science and technology to persons who are sick and suffering.

2

Searching

S. James Adelstein and Myra B. Ramos

When Daniel Tosteson accepted the call to become Dean of the Faculty of Medicine at Harvard University in 1977, he made it clear to faculty and administrators alike that reform of undergraduate medical education was high on his agenda. This should have come as no surprise, as he had a past record of great interest in the subject both at Duke University and, in the short time he spent as dean, at the University of Chicago. However, in their introduction to the faculty, probably all new deans of medical schools display an interest in the educational program(s), and such an interest is expected. In addition, although Harvard Medical School was not usually in the vanguard of American medical curricular reform, it was in the habit of picking up good practices from elsewhere and of making a few innovations of its own. For a new dean to act likewise, therefore, was not unanticipated. What was not anticipated was the extent of reform that the school would undertake. This chapter describes how the dean mobilized faculty interest in educational reform, engaged faculty groups in the planning process, secured faculty approval to move forward, developed funding, and utilized the experience of other schools.

Dean Tosteson faced a three-decade history of contentious shifts in the general medical curriculum. In the mid-1960s, following the experience of Western Reserve University, Harvard Medical School initiated an interdisciplinary first year that focused on cell and systems biology and a second year that emphasized pathophysiology by combining the elements of systematic pathology with laboratory medicine and clinical didactic teaching. Clerkships were offered in the third year, and a varied elective program in the fourth. The robust pathophysiology course also provided the basis of the Harvard—Massachusetts Institute of Technology Division of Health Sciences and Technology (HST) biomedical curriculum, leading to an M.D. degree. Offering clerkships in the third year accommodated an increasing demand for early specialty selection, but in the eyes of some faculty it also led to the premature handing over of education of medical students to house officers and residents. In 1965, in response to concern that the basic science departments might no longer have a rational place in the medical school, the interdisciplinary first year reverted to a group of basic science courses in anatomy, histology, biochemistry, physiology, neurobiology, microbiology, and pathology; these courses, however, which with one in pharmacology had previously occupied one and a half years in the curriculum, were now squeezed into a single academic year. The rationale for this compression was that some of the material (for example, systematic pathology) was now included in the pathophysiology course, and required material for the first-year courses was therefore reduced. This old wound would return to haunt the designers of the New Pathway curriculum, and compaction of the time allocated to the sciences basic to medicine remained a constant source of contention. (How the new biology led to a fear of extinction among basic science departments is a story of its own and has to do intellectually with the reductionism and convergence caused by molecular and cell biology. The threat to the departments was real, as evidenced by the organization of medical education within biological sciences at the University of Chicago and Brown University.)

This return to departmental hegemony in both preclinical and clinical courses led to a significant increase in the coursework required for graduation at the expense of elective time. As the course requirements mounted, faculty and students demanded some relief, and, as a result, graduation criteria were reduced to residency and distribution requirements; the only obligatory courses were Introduction to Clinical Medicine, a medicine clerkship (three months), a surgery clerkship (two months), and passing grades in Parts I and II of the National Board of Medical Examiners examination. A concentration requirement was instituted to ensure that all students would study something in depth, but it was not popular with students and was eliminated.

A strong advisory system guided students through the loose set of requirements. But in practice most students took the same courses for the first three years, and as a result the adviser's roles became chiefly those of proponent and guide. Because some of the selective core clerkships (for example, obstetrics and psychiatry) were less popular than others, members of the faculty who could not envision a medical degree without some experience in these specialties called for an expansion of the roster of required clerkships. This was the situation at Harvard Medical School when Dean Tosteson asked the faculty to address educational reform.

Generating Faculty Interest

Daniel Tosteson, upon becoming dean, recruited a group of deputy deans responsible for administrative and academic matters. The administrative deans oversaw administration, resources, and special projects; the academic deans oversaw academic programs, students and alumni, and hospital liaisons. To bring this diverse group together and develop a vision for the future course of the school, Tosteson held two decanal retreats. The first, in the winter of 1978, addressed primarily organizational matters; the second, in the summer of 1978, focused on how to sensitize the faculty to the need for reform, and profound reform at that, not merely tinkering with the calendar and the graduation requirements. To guide the discussion an options paper was prepared by a member of the dean's staff.

Of the several possibilities outlined in this paper, the most innovative suggestion was to divide students and faculty into groups to be designated as academic societies. These groups were to serve both as forums for the discussion of educational needs and as engines for major curricular innovations. During the 1978–79 academic year the Dean for Students and Alumni organized these societies, with distinguished senior faculty serving as masters. But although the societies did foster collegiality among students and faculty and their programs covered a broad range of medically relevant subjects, they did not take up or act on the subject of medical education in a substantive way.

Searching for other forums that could concentrate on educational issues, the Dean's Office organized a series of annual workshops and symposiums on education in general and on medical education in general. The workshops were internal dialogues among the medical school's students and faculty, while the symposiums brought in outside speakers to share their experience and give advice. The workshops were held in June 1979, April 1980, May 1981, and May 1982; the symposiums, in September 1979, December 1980, and January 1982.

At the 1979 workshop students, faculty, and house staff addressed the question "What do we want Harvard Medical School graduates to know how to do, and how does the learning environment foster or hinder the achievement of these goals?" Three-member panels composed of a faculty member, a student, and a house officer discussed individual papers distributed in advance. A number of problems and obstacles in the curriculum and learning environment were identified, including variability in the quality of teaching; diversity in styles of teaching; a relative paucity of senior faculty involvement in clinical teaching and a corresponding burden on the resident staff, who themselves were engaged in learning; an often undifferentiated mix of core learning material plus specialized faculty research interests; inadequate breadth of the required clinical clerkship experiences; lack of a conceptual framework for the frequently overwhelming amount of factual information presented; student anonymity (particularly in the first two years, but felt in clinical rotations as well); overreliance on the lecture format in the preclinical years; a tendency for examinations to emphasize rote recall rather than analytical thinking; and relative lack of articulation among the various segments of the curriculum.

Several recommendations emerged from the discussions: greater student participation in the learning process; fostering of faculty–student relationships with long-term continuity; greater engagement of senior faculty, particularly in clinical teaching; development of explicit educational objectives for all courses; identification by course and clerkship heads of core learning material and educational priorities; testing procedures that encourage conceptual thinking and form the basis for self-education; the establishment of workshops for the improvement of teaching; a critical approach to the medical literature and medical practice; increased use of small-group learning situations; greater emphasis on developing interpersonal skills; increased faculty incentives and awards for excellence in teaching; development of specific organizing principles to guide the establishment of curricular priorities and the allocation of scarce resources such as faculty and student time; improved intracurricular articulation, with attention to prerequisites and transitions; more emphasis on topics in behavioral science, preventive medicine, decision analysis, and biostatistics; and creation of a greater sense of community. The members of this workshop were prescient: all these recommendations and very few others became central goals of the New Pathway four years later.

During the next year four of these recommendations were addressed directly: a record of teaching experience was included in each faculty member's curriculum vitae to be used explicitly in the criteria for appointment and promotion; a committee was established to survey offerings in the quantitative, statistical sciences and to identify needs in this area, and a new course in decision theory was offered to third- and fourth-year students; a pilot project for the improvement of teaching skills was begun through the Harvard-Danforth Center for Teaching and Learning (now the Derek Bok Center); and the neurology clerkship was revised to increase faculty participation (students spent the entire first week with a faculty member learning to perform a neurologic examination, after which they joined the ward team).

The April 1980 workshop opened with a review of the year's progress and a reiteration of some important recommendations:

- There should be explicit rewards for teaching, in terms of both promotions and pay; on the other hand, allocation of some time to teaching is an intrinsic part of faculty duties.
- Senior faculty should be more fully engaged in clinical teaching.
- Competency-based criteria should be used for entry into the clinical clerkships.
- The student should be viewed as an apprentice going on to journeyman; thus, the preceptorship experience in defining the patient–doctor encounter should begin in the first year as part of a continuum extending through the clerkship experience.
- The abrupt transition from the first two years to the second two years should be eased, with more problem solving in the earlier period and less unsupervised problem resolution in the latter.
- The isolation and belittling of students caused by passive learning should be reduced.

Three general topics were discussed at the workshop. The first involved the benefits of small-group learning: a small group would be more stimulating than lectures and large-group conferences and would engage the skills of analysis, criticism, and discrimination that students bring to medical school; students would learn early to articulate questions and answers to a small, attentive, and critical audience; small classes would allow for diversity of experience and interest and greater interaction; small-group preclinical teaching could be more difficult but also more interesting and challenging than the lecture-intensive mode.

The second topic concerned critical approaches to medical information and the medical literature. The following points were made: because the medical school experience is a mix of scholarly and professional learning, a knowledgeable faculty group could be asked to define the basic knowledge, skills, and attitudes required of all students; students look to the faculty for direction as they seek an approach to a vast array of information; students should seek understanding rather than learn facts—the payoff of self-enlightenment is self-education; the faculty should be concerned less with teaching content and more with teaching how to set priorities in assimilating facts; and the computer should be used more frequently as an interactive and responsive tool for learning and information retrieval.

Last, the workshop dealt with the development of procedures for student evaluation that would encourage conceptual thinking and self-education. In response to the concern that course heads sometimes did not transmit the goals of their courses, and thus left unclear what would be emphasized in examinations, suggestions included varying the examination format to involve analysis and integration as well as recall, making self-assessment and self-pacing available, and improving feedback to students about progress and level of mastery.

The May 1981 workshop focused in greater detail on the evaluation of student performance. The participants offered four perspectives. These were evaluation as threshold: defining and determining a satisfactory level of performance; evaluation as diagnosis: providing feedback for self-improvement; evaluation as recommendation: describing student performance and attributes for internship applications; and evaluation as curricular diagnosis: using student performance as a measure of teaching success. The second and fourth concerns recurred throughout the development of the New Pathway project.

Like the workshops, the symposiums dealt with educational issues but added the perspectives of outside speakers. The first, in September 1979, dealt with three topics: the impact of education on the student; the content of medical education; and methods of learning and teaching. Samuel Bloom of Mount Sinai Medical School addressed the issue of socialization among medical students. He faulted Harvard and other research-intensive medical schools for producing "frontiersmen," independent solo practitioners and scientists. He encouraged the inclusion of social issues in the curriculum and a definition of the physician's role in addressing them. Alexander Astin of the Graduate School of Education at the University of California at Los Angeles also examined how institutions influence the behavior of students. His studies indicated that institutions exert little or no influence in the cognitive realm but may influence affective behavior, and that in this respect the most significant variable is student identification with the academic community. Small size is important, as is anything that favors social interaction among students and faculty members, such as special tracks, clubs, athletic facilities, and local organizations.

Another speaker, Paul Beeson, an experienced and respected medical educator, had made a systematic study of the Harvard Medical School course catalogue and had come to the following conclusions: organized ambulatory clinical teaching was absent and should not be; many of the elective offerings were too narrow and too technical, and the elective period should be used for more substantial matters; too little time was devoted to the humanities and the behavioral and social sciences; and students should be encouraged to pursue research throughout medical school.

John Evans and Victor Neufeld, initiators of the reform in medical education that accompanied the establishment of the McMaster Medical School, discussed the advantages of interdepartmental, problem-oriented teaching, which avoids the shortcomings of departmental single-discipline courses: a tendency to increase the already excessive information overload; difficulty in adding new areas, which could only be inserted in small chunks; and unresolved arguments over the necessary core. Evans and Neufeld had adopted a process-oriented approach in the belief that content would follow: if students were more self-directed and more active in their own learning, they would be better prepared for the necessity of continuing self-education. They recommended increased faculty–student and student–student interaction, working in small groups, and maintaining continuity. The speakers also stressed the need to separate the educational program from the management of the individual departments. The McMaster

M.D. program has its own manager and steering committee. Furthermore, faculty members are expected to spend an average of 20 percent of their time in the program, and participation is strongly considered in faculty promotion. Evans emphasized that central administrative control of the program was essential to its continued success.

The December 1980 symposium was concerned with information overload and information management in medical education and medical practice. Thomas Allen of the Massachusetts Institute of Technology and Louis Robinson of International Business Machines discussed gatekeeping and technology, respectively. Jill Larkin of the Carnegie-Mellon Institute described the differences between experts and novices in their approaches to solving problems. Jack Myers of the University of Pittsburgh and Eugene Stead of Duke University outlined their own efforts to develop expert systems for medical diagnosis. Eugene Garfield of the Institute for Scientific Information and Kenneth Warren of the Rockefeller Foundation recommended combining the use of computers with a systematic approach to solving overload problems and accessing the current literature. The presentations stirred a sympathetic response from the participating faculty. The late Norman Geschwind, chairman of the Harvard Medical School Curriculum Committee and an expert on higher cognitive function, made an appeal to avoid cerebral technological obsolescence, by which he meant overreliance on the human memory, and asked that modern technology "free us from intellectual drudgery." Octo Barnett, director of the Laboratory of Computer Science at the Massachusetts General Hospital, asked that students learn more about decision making and utilize that skill in conjunction with expert systems. Arnold Relman, editor of the *New England Journal of Medicine,* reiterated the need to access the medical literature by machine while critically reading it with a prepared mind.

The final symposium, in January 1982, focused on the discontinuities between college and medical school and between medical school and residency training. Participants discussed some of the baleful effects of being a premedical student, as well as the overlaps between general medical education and specialty residency training. However, no specific consensus emerged, and the interface issues remained contentious and unresolved at the inception of the New Pathway reform.

The workshop held in May 1982 was a milestone. The dean proposed launching a demonstration program involving twenty-five first-year students that would address four elements not handled adequately in the education of physicians:

- Commitment—respect and care for others, fostered further during medical education
- Cognitive style—emphasis on solving problems and finding information through use of modern technology
- Content—explicit and precise definition of the general knowledge base for all facets of medicine
- Continuity—more coherent planning for the entire sequence of medical education in college, medical school, and residency

He proposed a seven-year course of study characterized by

- Close personal relationships between students and faculty, fostered by working together in small groups
- A shared educational experience during half of scheduled instruction time, characterized by problem-solving through the case method and by self-learning and self-assessment using interactive, computer-assisted, audiovisual devices
- Interweaving of the arts and sciences basic to medicine with the clinical arts and sciences throughout the curriculum
- Acquisition of quantitative skills to gather and analyze quantitative clinical data
- A thesis requiring independent study

The response was mixed. Most respondents agreed that medical education needed a prod, but several disagreed with the dean's prescription for change. By and large there was agreement about the need to address commitment, cognitive style, and content, much less so about continuity. There was moderate enthusiasm about the use of case-study-based, problem-solving small groups, interweaving clinical and basic arts and sciences, and acquisition of quantitative analytical skills. The notion of a seven-year course of study that would overlap with college and residency training was not popular. Nonetheless, participants in the workshop overwhelmingly encouraged the dean to undertake a planning process, and several members of the faculty volunteered to be part of it.

These workshops and symposiums, each involving about 100 students and faculty sequestered off-campus for a full day, were instrumental in raising the consciousness of faculty and students about problems with the current form of medical education, in beginning conversations about how the form might be changed, and in identifying faculty most interested in undergraduate medical education and its improvement. Away from distractions, they mobilized interest, gave the subject legitimacy, and created a forum for launching a new program. Moreover, the discussions during the working sessions and meals fostered collegial relationships that proved important for the planning and implementation process. Unfortunately, although invitations for the workshops and symposiums were widely distributed, the same faculty members tended to attend. As a result, certain key faculty, especially department heads, did not participate in any or many of the discussions and consequently remained unaware of developments. They had to be informed separately, and many remained skeptical about or actively opposed to the project. In retrospect, we realize that we should have worked harder to include a somewhat broader group in these preliminary colloquiums.

Planning

After the May 1982 workshop Dean Tosteson appointed a planning group of students and faculty charged with drafting a statement of objectives and a curricular plan for the demonstration project. In September the Josiah Macy, Jr., Foundation provided a grant to support planning activities. The Planning Committee, chaired by Dean Tosteson, consisted of other administrators (Daniel Federman, James Adelstein, Myra Ramos); natural scientists (Edwin Furshpan, Philip Leder); social scientists (Robert Coles, Leon Eisenberg); clinicians, including three department heads and a hospital president (Judah Folkman, Robert Moellering, John Potts, Mitchell Rabkin, William Silen, Thomas Smith, Arnold Weinberg); students (Lisa Guay-Woodford, Paul Unger, Herbert Virgin); and two faculty members chosen for their special competencies, an expert in the case-study method from the Graduate School of Business Administration (C. Roland Christensen) and an expert in medical informatics (Octo Barnett).

This planning group met at least twice a month. At midyear it circulated an interim report to the entire faculty for comment. Its basic elements were those elaborated in the dean's proposal to the May 1982 workshop. It set forth a demonstration project to address the entire span of general medical education: a seven-year program that would include the last two years of college and the first year of residency training; a single faculty group to develop the curriculum; a learning environment that would emphasize close student–faculty contact, small groups and tutorials, self-learning and self-assessment, analytic and problem-solving activities, case discussions, interactive computer programs and the use of information technology, and independent study. The interim report was discussed in meetings of the Curriculum Committee, the Faculty Council, the Committee of Professors, and the Conference of Department Heads; it was also the subject of written responses. Again, the reaction was mixed. Generally, there was little opposition to a demonstration project that involved the usual four years of medical school. Most of the opposition related to extending the responsibility of the Faculty of Medicine to the college years (perceived to be an intrusion into the preprofessional school experience) and of the medical school into residency training (perceived to be the domain of hospital-based specialists). Preclinical faculty, both in departments whose teaching loads were relatively light and in those, such as the Department of Anatomy and Cellular Biology, whose loads were already heavy, were worried that the proposed program would increase the teaching demands by running two tracks. It was the latter concern that was later responsible, in part, for an early expansion from pilot project to schoolwide program. The Planning Committee dealt with concerns about infringements on undergraduate college by recommending that the issue be discussed separately with members of the Faculty of Arts and Sciences. (A group was convened for this purpose, again under the sponsorship of the Macy Foundation, but it moved at a slower pace and developed a different set of objectives.)

In early 1983 the Planning Committee established three broad-based working groups of faculty and students to write goals for attitudes and professional characteristics, for skills, and for knowledge. The working groups produced thoughtful sets of objectives under each of the following categories:

- Attitudes toward
  - patients and colleagues
  - society at large
  - learning
  - one's self
- Skills in
  - acquiring information from and about patients
  - obtaining, retrieving, and storing information

working effectively with one's peers and the health team
communicating effectively with patients, families, and colleagues
performing basic diagnostic procedures
problem-solving
self-awareness

- Knowledge as an understanding of
  the patient as a living being
  the patient as an individual and as a social being
  the principles of prevention and therapeutic strategies
  the statistical and probabilistic aspects of human biology and clinical medicine
  the complex texture of knowledge and the importance of detail, achieved in part through in-depth study of a particular subject

In May 1983 the New Pathway Planning Committee presented its report to the Curriculum Committee, the Faculty Council, and then to the Faculty of Medicine at large. The report attempted to reassure those who were concerned about the possible effect on the school's resources by stipulating that the program would be "financed by external sources of support." For those who desired data on which to base any future decisions regarding extension of the pilot track or its elements, it also provided that the program would be "evaluated by quantitative and qualitative measures."

A number of Curriculum Committee members had reservations—for opposite reasons—about establishing a demonstration project. Those who supported the proposed innovation were concerned that its benefits would not be immediately available to all students. Those who were apprehensive about the new approach were alarmed by the dean's clearly stated intent that the new program be a model for extension rather than a permanent separate track; would authorization of a pilot constitute a "blank check," placing future events beyond their control? This double hurdle was surmounted by an implementation resolution submitted by Harvey Goldman (who became Faculty Dean for Medical Education in 1987) and approved by the Curriculum Committee. The resolution endorsed the introduction of a new pathway for medical education for up to twenty-five students from each class beginning in the fall of 1985; the curricular goals described in the New Pathway Planning Committee report; the establishment of a new academic society to carry out the new program; and the seeking of outside financial support. Crucial to gaining Curriculum Committee acceptance, the resolution further stipulated that a group of faculty and students be identified "to design and develop a specific program, with the understanding that the Curriculum Committee will review each segment of the curriculum; and to provide a plan for applying successful components of the new pathway to a larger segment of the medical school class."

Before the report was considered by the full Faculty of Medicine, representatives of the New Pathway Planning Committee, including Dean Federman, had attended meetings with the preclinical departments in which skepticism had been greatest. Although the concerns about faculty time were only somewhat assuaged at these meetings and the efficiency and efficacy of self-directed learning were challenged, as was the concept of case-based problem-solving in the basic sciences, the faculty agreed to allow the planning process to continue so long as the plan came back to them for final approval. In particular, some faculty members wanted a more detailed accounting of the material to be taught, how it was to be presented, and what the demands would be on faculty time.

Over the summer of 1983 members of the Dean's Office discussed how to transform the New Pathway Planning Committee report into a curricular plan for twenty-five students who were to enter in the fall of 1985 as an academic unit to be called the Oliver Wendell Holmes Society. Two retreats of interested faculty advanced the process. In the first, it was agreed that each curricular segment should be integrated both across disciplines and between basic and clinical sciences. In the second, a working structure to develop the curriculum was approved. This included a Steering Committee (successor to the Planning Committee) to oversee the planning effort and assume responsibility for policy decisions. Eight interdisciplinary curricular design groups were charged with developing specific curricular segments, which were intentionally given names symbolizing the newness of approach (for example, The Patient, Identity and Defense, and Information Processing and Behavior). A Curriculum Coordinating Committee comprising the head of every curricular design group was established to achieve continuity, completeness, and integration; and support committees were named to develop resources and personnel in specific areas such as educational methods, information technology, faculty development, and program evaluation. How these groups proceeded, racing the clock so that a first group of students could matriculate by the fall of 1985, is described in Chapter 3.

Faculty Approval

During 1983 and 1984 the New Pathway planners reported often to the Curriculum Committee. In the January 1984 intersession period, a problem-based course using tutorials and clinical problem cases was organized by Jeffrey Berman, the first of many students to take a year off from studies to work on New Pathway medical education. The thirteen first-year student participants and the pilot-course faculty were unanimously enthusiastic about the approach.

The progress report presented to the Curriculum Committee in April 1984 sketched broad content outlines of the curriculum and presented an implementation timetable. General scheduling guidelines specified that the total number of classroom hours for the shared portion (60 percent) of the curriculum would not exceed fifteen per week, with no more than one lecture per day. Educational methods were to "promote active learning, questioning, problem-solving, and critical thinking" with an emphasis on experiential and problem-based learning.

Discussion of the New Pathway plan at the April 1984 Curriculum Committee meeting revealed considerable apprehension about the emphasis on problem-based learning, the proposed omission of psychiatry as a required clerkship, and the potential "loss of disciplines as disciplines" exemplified by the interdisciplinary basic science blocks. In response, the New Pathway Steering Committee drew up a policy statement reaffirming the commitment to problem-based learning in combination with other educational methods (including "a limited number of lectures") but also promising to consult with the departments about content development.

At its May 1984 meeting the Curriculum Committee expressed concern about the potential loss of control implied by approval of the progress report. Nevertheless the committee voted to accept the report with the understanding that it would continue to receive periodic reports on details of the program and would later review their conformance with requirements for graduation from Harvard Medical School.

With this acceptance of the pedagogical philosophy, design principles, and curricular organization, planning for specific courses could proceed. In January 1985 the Curriculum Committee reviewed planning materials for the first semester of the New Pathway project; in May it heard presentation of course materials for the second semester. In subsequent years it would review plans for second-year course blocks as well as for each of the newly designed New Pathway core clerkships.

Funding

A commitment had been made to fund the new program from external sources. A grant from the Josiah Macy, Jr., Foundation provided seed money for planning activities during 1983–84, including the two faculty retreats and the work of the curricular design groups. The American Medical International Foundation and the Arthur Vining Davis Foundations were also early contributors. Subsequent gifts were received from the R. H. Macy Foundation, the Exxon Educational Foundation, and individual donors, including Harvard alumni. The Hewlett Packard Company made a $5 million grant of computer equipment and software development support over a five-year period. In the fall of 1985 the Kaiser Family Foundation awarded a $3 million grant that assured the first three years of implementation and supported, in particular, program evaluation, content on health promotion and disease prevention, and diffusion of the results of the project. An additional $1 million from the Kaiser Family Foundation in 1988 supported extension of the pilot program to the entire school and development of the clinical curriculum in particular.

The Role of Other Institutions

With their presentation of the pioneering McMaster University curriculum at our 1979 educational symposium, John Evans and Victor Neufeld greatly stimulated our interest in the potential of student-centered and problem-based learning. On several subsequent visits, Neufeld offered advice and encouragement based on his extensive experience. Our initial thinking about faculty development also benefited greatly from a meeting with a team of faculty from the problem-based Primary Care Curriculum (PCC) at the University of New Mexico. Jeffrey Berman, the Harvard medical student who organized the prototypic tutorial course, was one of many New Pathway project staff and faculty who visited both the McMaster and the PCC programs. A faculty planning retreat featured a keynote speaker from Southern Illinois University's problem-based track. Through frequent communication and exchange with these schools as well as with Mercer University, Rush University Medical School, and the universities of Limburg and Newcastle, we increased our understanding of the task we had set ourselves. The resulting program at Harvard Medical School, tailored to the local culture and opportunities for innovation, is a "hybrid," drawing both on new approaches and on traditional strengths.

3

Strategies for Change

Gordon T. Moore

Guided by the dean's conception, the subcommittees working on the new curriculum identified the parameters of change. The New Pathway would mark a fundamental shift in the way Harvard Medical School students were taught. It was eventually to include all students and to span all four years. The new educational approach would challenge students to be more actively involved in defining what they learned and how they learned it, moving from a passive and teacher-directed experience toward one in which they were actively engaged in thinking and learning. The curriculum was to provide a general education common to all students rather than emphasize any one career such as research, subspecialty medicine, or primary care. Basic sciences and clinical medicine were to be interwoven throughout the curriculum. Similar integration was planned for the behavioral, social, and natural sciences, and boundaries between disciplines and departments in teaching were to be substantially decreased. The curriculum would be designed and delivered as an organic whole from the perspective of a single faculty looking at the entire span of general medical education. Most of the Harvard faculty, though supporting these general educational goals, were by no means in agreement about the specifics. Many felt the medical school curriculum had undergone several revisions during the previous quarter-century. Some expressed concern that the faculty would not be adequately motivated for such a wholesale alteration in teaching methods and content. Inadequate finances, lack of academic recognition, and competing research priorities were raised as important practical issues to be solved before moving ahead.

The New Pathway planners knew that moving from general principles to an operating program would be difficult. They recognized the importance of having a well-conceived strategy for getting started, including defining goals, identifying means to achieve those goals, developing policies and procedures, finding appropriate funding and personpower to achieve the desired ends, and developing plans to identify how to overcome logistical and political barriers.

The strategic plan for the New Pathway project was designed to stimulate and protect innovation, encourage interdisciplinary integration and collective oversight for the entire curriculum, and enhance project management. The major elements included the creation of an experimental parallel track; the use of central planning groups to develop shared values and vision for the innovation and to integrate the curriculum so that learning objectives were systematic and redundancies minimized; a managerial orientation to the planning and implementation process, including the use of a program budget, a detailed timetable and task lists, and the rapid development of a centralized staff of professional educators to assist in all aspects of operational development; and a plan to reduce barriers.

Creating an Experimental Separate Track

One of the most important steps was to initiate the new curriculum as a separate, experimental track. This strategy was aimed at overcoming the resistance of many faculty members to significant change in the curriculum. In the prior twenty-five years the faculty had instituted perhaps a half-dozen relatively small changes in the curriculum. Almost all involved the entire medical school class. This experience persuaded those planning the New Pathway that the compromises necessary to initiate schoolwide changes in the curriculum would considerably weaken the degree of innovation, and that the only way to achieve far-reaching change would be to start with a volunteer subset of students and faculty. Using a separate track would make it possible to approach the innovation as an experiment and to encourage radical thinking, to attract the relatively small number of faculty who were dissatisfied with the traditional curriculum and excited about the prospect of change, and to enroll voluntarily students who welcomed a different educational approach. These factors allowed the planning process to be as creative as possible.

An important benefit of the separate track was the pioneering spirit and enthusiasm generated by a small, tight-knit group of faculty and students. The creation of such a collegial group was a long-term objective. From the outset of the planning for the new curriculum, the dean emphasized his hope that each of the school's academic societies would personalize a generic curricular approach and enhance the relationship among students, among faculty, and between teachers and their students.

The Curriculum Committee approved the general principles of the new curriculum and its inception as a separate track, and was kept informed of progress, reviewing each component as it was developed. The experimental status of the project and the continuation of the traditional courses and teaching format predisposed the committee to be tolerant and supportive, although it also voiced criticisms. The fact that the committee was not involved with details of the prototype design of the new curriculum shielded the innovation and created the freedom to design and implement without a cumbersome and detailed approval process.

Designing the curriculum as a separate track had another expected benefit: it created a sense of excitement, and even of competition, about curricular methods. Having two curriculums, each with its own avid supporters, stimulated each group to do its best. As the shape of the new curriculum emerged, faculty engaged in lively discussion about the strengths and weaknesses of each approach. These discussions were formalized by periodic workshops on topics related to the educational changes under way. Many faculty members found the sense of competition between the two student and faculty groups at once stimulating and distressing. Although this energy sometimes got out of hand, it probably improved efforts in both the new and the traditional curriculums during the development and early stages of implementation of the New Pathway project.

Protecting the innovation was important, but the separate track was never conceived as a permanent second pathway for medical education. Rather, it was envisioned as a way to pilot new ideas, to determine which were most effective in our setting, and to use this information to design a final single curriculum for all medical students. Because the ultimate goal was faculty approval of the concepts underlying the new curriculum, the planners encouraged open communication so that faculty would understand and, ultimately, support the innovations. First, interested faculty were given the opportunity to join the group of planners, and department heads were invited to designate key faculty to lead and participate in the New Pathway program. Second, each department was asked to designate a liaison between the department, which was responsible for supplying faculty to teach the new curriculum, and the planning groups responsible for designing the educational program. Third, the new program reported frequently on its progress to the Curriculum Committee and to a special Steering Committee chaired by Dean Tosteson, which met monthly to review important decisions and to monitor progress. This committee included influential members of the faculty, some of whom were skeptical about the new approach to education. Later, faculty development programs brought interested faculty together and communicated reactions to the new curriculum and tips for teaching to each succeeding faculty group.

Central Planning Groups

For logistical reasons, the curriculum had to be divided into self-contained courses of ten to twelve weeks each. Each block was deliberately interdisciplinary, generally comprising two or three of the traditional disciplines. The New Pathway planners sought a faculty leader to direct the planning and teaching of each block. These leaders had emerged from the dean's planning meetings, at which interested faculty had signaled their support by participating in preliminary working groups. Thus, when the time came to implement the new track, there was already a group of faculty from different departments who were prepared to participate or who could be instrumental in finding other colleagues to take over for them.

Each block of the preclinical and clinical curriculum was developed, designed, and delivered by a curricular design group chaired by a single faculty leader who had broad disciplinary and teaching experience. Scientists and clinicians from the multiple disciplines involved in the curricular block collaborated to design and develop their course materials, with special emphasis on developing cases for use in problem-based teaching.

To achieve a balanced and integrated educational program, a single faculty group needed to plan, design, provide oversight, and implement the overall course of study. The head of each of the curricular design groups joined the New Pathway staff in an interlocking directorate that became known as the Curriculum Coordinating Committee. This multidisciplinary group met often and regularly to coordinate development of the curriculum and to develop policies and procedures. It reached agreement about gaps and redundancies in content and experiences as well as trade-offs required to fit the entire curriculum into the allotted calendar.

Managing the Development of the Curriculum

The New Pathway director assembled a core project staff consisting of administrative and support staff as well as experts in curriculum development and faculty training. Each year a new medical student fellow joined the New Pathway staff, which was further supplemented by several faculty members with a special interest in medical education. The dominant activity of this staff was to assist each curricular design group in developing the blocks of courses that made up the four-year curriculum. The staff of professional educators functioned in a matrix with the curricular design groups, providing administrative and educational support, while integrating the work of each curricular design group into the overall plan for the development of the curriculum.

The entire development process was complex and required careful management. Early on, faculty discussion groups had specified important general parameters such as the balance of time between electives and required courses and the frequency of lectures (limited to one per day), and had developed general statements of purpose about the lectures and how they would relate to problem-based learning. The Curriculum Coordinating Committee, acting on staff recommendations, identified further specific and tangible products to be achieved and devised a timetable for doing so. Once specific planning had begun, these and other specifications helped design groups to work semi-independently while relying on clear guidelines about what was to be included and how the course was to be taught.

Having these "building blocks" focused the actions of all parties on concrete outcomes. In the curricular development process, for example, a specified set of case materials was designated for each problem, and the educational staff and faculty heads for each block were expected to develop a course book consisting of a description of the material to be covered, general course objectives, and the set of problems for that block. In addition, we developed a program guide that described the reasons for the new curriculum, the theory underpinning the educational approaches we used, the general objectives, and problem-based learning methodology. A fourth-year student on leave to work as a fellow with the project developed a student guide to problem-based learning. The Director of Faculty Development initiated a series of educational exercises about problem-based learning, made suggestions about how to improve lecturing, and described other educational approaches that might be used in both the traditional and the new curriculums.

Equally important were modifications in administrative support procedures. For the first time, to support the New Pathway project a detailed educational program budget was developed to identify milestones and the resources needed to reach them. A funding campaign approached potential outside sources of support and obtained several grants to develop different aspects of the new program. Each award provided an opportunity to describe the project both inside and outside the medical school and to create a sense of momentum for it.

In 1984 plans for a new educational facility commenced. The funding campaign and the design of a facility specifically suited to problem-based learning focused considerable attention on this method both within and outside the faculty.

Perhaps the most important element of the strategy was the goal-directed management of the entire process to guide production and keep it on schedule. Strong central management was needed to balance the heavy commitment to discussion and review by faculty and the decentralized development of the curricular blocks. Business-related techniques such as program budgeting, strategic planning, use of critical path methods to specify milestones and develop timetables, and project monitoring to assure progress were valuable tools in managing people and projects.

The early, explicit commitment to having the curriculum ready by the fall of 1985 provided a practical focus and minimized discussion of theoretical issues. The general approach emphasized building the curriculum and then fixing what did not work on the basis of experience running the new curriculum. Deadlines focused debate and forced planners to identify alternative options and make decisions quickly.

Reducing Barriers

At the start of the project, the steering group recognized that faculty resistance and lack of money, space, time, and academic recognition could block curricular change. All the resources of the Dean's Office were directed toward minimizing the effect of these barriers. The program's budget included use of supplemental financing to secure a modest but separate space. This also allowed the project to develop its identity early. The use of limited amounts of money provided recognition of the extra effort of busy faculty. Further, a special task force specified ways to document excellence in teaching and to use this information in the academic promotion process. Procedures to evaluate faculty teaching activities were instituted on a trial basis starting in 1985. This effort served as a precursor to schoolwide use of teacher-clinician criteria for promotion in 1988.

General Principles

A handful of principles emerged from the experience of implementing problem-based learning at Harvard Medical School, including:

- The importance of a strategy to isolate and protect the initial development of an educational innovation.
- The need to counterbalance the decentralized financial and operational organization of most medical schools. To achieve comprehensive curricular change, a centralized, interdisciplinary group must provide oversight and integration of the entire span of medical education.
- The importance of balancing freedom to experiment and faculty participation through evaluation, review, and comment. Recognizing and using the creative energy and commitment of students and faculty interested in adopting new approaches involve not derailing their effort by forcing them to work with nay-sayers. Dividing functions and authority among the faculty achieves this goal. Although the whole faculty needs to assent to the overarching goals and purposes of education, operational implementation can

be confined to a relatively small group of planners and workers. While all faculty members are encouraged to review and comment, authority for important detailed decisions must be reserved to smaller groups or to individuals.
- The value of using management techniques to facilitate the design, development, and production of the curriculum.
- The utility of staff support to complement the efforts of faculty.

4

The First Curriculum: Content and Process

Gordon T. Moore

Approximately one year before the projected starting date in the fall of 1985, the Curriculum Committee approved the pilot curriculum for student volunteers numbering up to one-fifth of the incoming class. The general characteristics of this curriculum emerged from a complicated process of discussion stimulated by subcommittee reports, outside visitors, suggestions from the Dean's Office, and educational workshops.

The new curriculum sought to change both the form and the content of general medical education. The skills and attitudes that underlie effective learning and thinking were acknowledged to be as important as the specific knowledge acquired. Science was clearly the language of medicine, but the lasting elements of medical education were viewed as the capacity for scientific thinking and not merely the body of particular scientific facts existing in the different fields of medicine at any point in time. The New Pathway curriculum sought to exercise the student's capacity to think and to discover while also ensuring that facts were learned.

Starting from the premise that responsibility for learning lies with the student, the designers of the new curriculum sought to make the learning process challenging and deeply satisfying. They sought to design an educational process that guided, stimulated, and challenged, rather than directed. They aspired to create a society of learners committed to reflection on the learning process as well as on the outcome of that process. They conceived of medical school as the beginning of a lifelong process of self-education. Converting this general philosophy into an actual curriculum was a formidable challenge.

Defining the Features of the Curriculum

Many types of educational methods were to be used in the New Pathway project, including lectures, seminars, laboratories, hands-on skills training, and computer-assisted learning. But the central educational method for the new curriculum became problem-based learning.[1] In this method, pioneered at McMaster University Medical School, students analyze carefully written clinical (or, less frequently, research) cases in tutorial groups facilitated by a faculty leader. The students discuss the case, hypothesize about what is going on, and identify learning tasks for independent study. In independent self-directed study, students select the learning approach that works best for them, including standard textbooks, original literature, correlated laboratory or computer exercises, consultation with expert faculty, and other approaches. In follow-up tutorial sessions, scheduled for several hours three times a week, students return to discuss what they have learned and to reformulate their learning objectives for another round of independent study. In this cycle, the tutorial serves as a forum for analyzing the case, setting learning agendas, discussing and elaborating what students learned during independent study, and refining and elaborating their knowledge. This is where students learn to work together. Most of the content learning takes place outside the tutorial.

This approach, based on adult learning theory, casts the student in the role of an active, responsible participant in the education process. We like this method for other reasons, as well:

- The discovery process—the quest to explain observations that are not fully understood—is at the heart of scientific inquiry. As students grapple with problems in their tutorial groups, they develop and practice problem-solving skills directly applicable to their future medical practice and scientific endeavors.
- Active engagement with the learning process is intellectually stimulating and powerfully motivating for students and faculty alike.
- Knowledge gained in the context in which it will be used is more likely to be recalled when needed. By studying the basic sciences to elucidate a relevant problem, students should find that knowledge more readily available when it is needed later.

- Emphasis is on the skills of independent learning. In the rapidly expanding world of biomedical knowledge, knowing how to continue learning after the completion of one's formal education is as important as the mastery of a body of current concepts and skills.
- The use of carefully selected problems encourages the students to integrate knowledge across diverse disciplines and fields.
- A learning contract between student and peers and between student and teacher is established in tutorial groups, creating an open commitment to a common goal and motivation to do the work.
- Group discussion fosters communication and acquisition of interpersonal skills needed for future work with colleagues and patients.

Reduced Scheduled Time

For problem-based learning and independent study methods to work, students require unscheduled time. Because we expected students to do a higher proportion of their work in self-directed independent study, we substantially reduced the amount of time allotted for lectures, seminars, and laboratory exercises. In the first year, for example, student–faculty contact time in the New Pathway curriculum was at least 40 percent less than in the traditional curriculum (Figure 4.1). Faculty-directed activities were restricted to the mornings, leaving all but one afternoon free for independent study or electives.

One Lecture a Day

The planning group endorsed limiting lectures to one per day, reasoning that too many lectures would compete for students' time and erode their impetus to direct their own learning. The lectures were intended to explicate difficult material, emphasize key concepts and principles, introduce unique disciplinary perspectives that could not be readily obtained through reading or independent study, and provide an organizational structure on which to build new learning. We hoped that the lecturers would particularly focus on helping students understand and put into a conceptual context the problems they encountered in self-directed learning. The best lecturers, it was reasoned, would sit in on tutorials and then relate their lectures to the students' areas of difficulty. Several lectures would be given by the

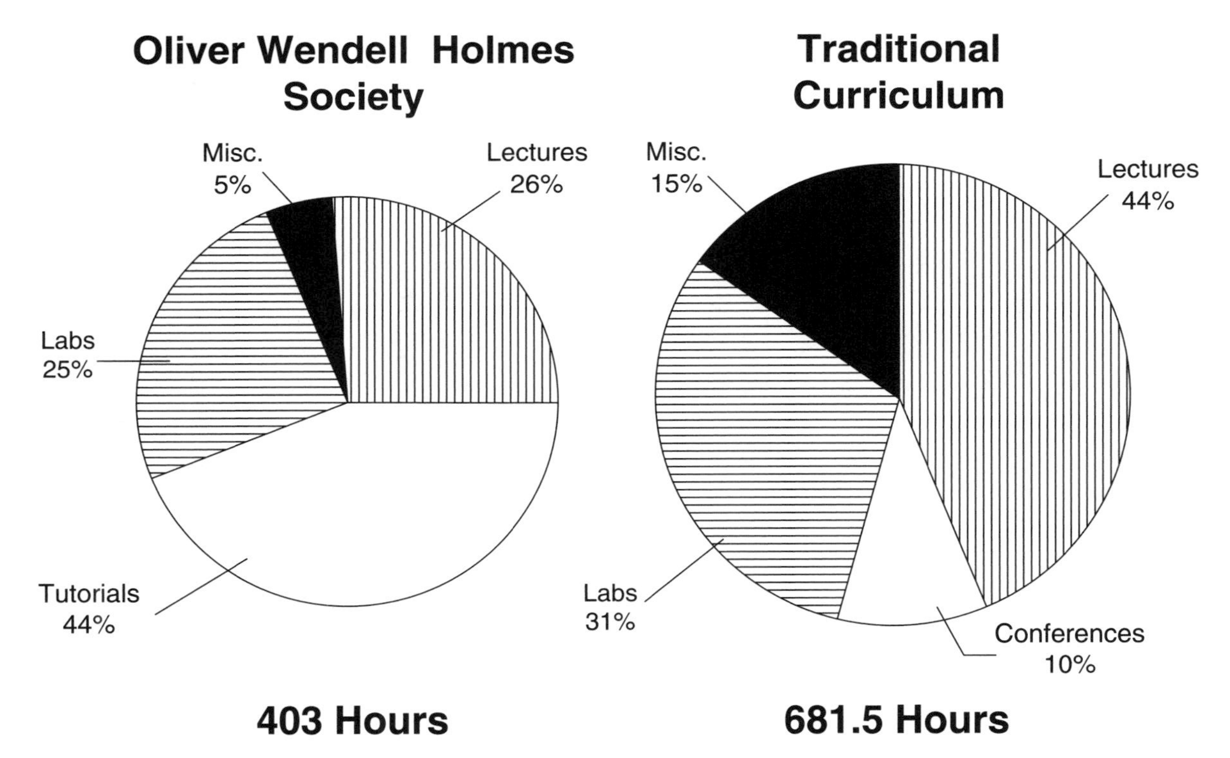

Figure 4.1 Student–faculty contact time in the New Pathway and traditional curriculums

same faculty member so that important topics could be presented in depth. Each faculty member was responsible, in the best of circumstances, for a minimum of four or five lectures.

Clinical and Basic Science Integration

Early clinical exposure created motivation and gave relevance to the preclinical curriculum. However, several basic science faculty members were worried that less time was now allotted for learning the scientific basis of medicine. The planners argued that any displacement of basic science would be counterbalanced by integrating science into the clinical curriculum. Moreover, the importance of science to medicine was to be reinforced by a required return to basic science in the last year of medical school.

The continued interrelationship between the basic and clinical sciences was a conceptual cornerstone of the curriculum. Early clinical correlation with basic science was a way to stimulate students to learn science and to develop a clinical context that might facilitate the recall of scientific concepts later on. For example, students might learn the rudiments of the chest examination at the time they discussed a pulmonary case and were carrying out gross and histological analysis of the lung. The relevance of the anatomy and histology was evident, and the clinical context provided cues for the students to recall what they had learned. Theoretically, students would use their own clinical cases during the third and fourth years to re-explore scientific principles and pathophysiology. The science reprise and, hopefully, an independent project would provide further opportunity for returning to explore a field in greater scientific depth.

The Patient–Doctor Concept

Written clinical cases served as the starting point for natural science learning, but we recognized that in their eagerness to learn the "hard" sciences students and faculty might be likely to defer or entirely omit studying and discussing social and behavioral concepts. Consequently, we wanted to create a course that would explore the patient–doctor relationship from the perspectives of history, sociology, anthropology, ethics, medical humanities, and the behavioral sciences while also introducing students to the clinical skills of interviewing and physical examination. As students learned clinical skills, they would also learn the principles of health promotion and disease prevention.

This thinking led to the development of a course called the Patient–Doctor in which students would begin in the first weeks of medical school to interview and examine patients. The instructional sequence was developed to coincide with biological, behavioral, and social science objectives. Issues of preventive and social medicine were tightly structured into the curriculum to correspond with relevant case discussions and patient experiences. This course interspersed clinical experiences involving real patients with large-group seminars and tutorial group discussions. Case presentations and videotapes were used as the focus for tutorial discussion, and students were expected to prepare for these discussions through assigned weekly readings. In contrast to the tutorial groups for problem-based learning, in which membership changed in each new block, the Patient–Doctor tutorial groups retained the same faculty and students throughout the three years of weekly meetings.

Learning Objectives

It quickly became clear that there was major tension between student-directed learning and the faculty's desire for systematic coverage of the disciplines and knowledge students needed to acquire. If students were free to select all their topics, their knowledge of medicine might be haphazard and nonrigorous. We quickly identified a number of approaches to minimize this problem, among them extensive specification of learning objectives across the curriculum, careful case selection, vertical integration, and training and guidance for tutors.

The most important element in assuring that students would learn what the faculty considered essential was to begin to think in terms of learning objectives rather than in terms of courses or lectures. Using course syllabuses from the traditional curriculum, we tried to determine the major learning objectives by analyzing the lectures and exercises. Next we made a rough allocation of learning objectives to each block. In the Curriculum Coordinating Committee, we eliminated important redundancies, resolved jurisdictional disputes between blocks, and identified major learning objectives not covered in the traditional curriculum. For example, a set of objectives related to life stages, which had not been explicitly covered in the traditional course work, became a major part of one of the courses in the New Pathway curriculum.

We developed a set of functional learning objectives that included preventive, behavioral, social, and population medicine as well as the biological sciences. Although students might not choose to study each of these areas in every tutorial case, we believed that recognizing the recurrence of these issues in cases throughout the curriculum would teach students the importance of these domains of learning when they were specifically addressed later.

As the curriculum grew, it became more difficult for the project staff to keep track of objectives and cases. Consequently, we developed a computer-based catalogue of cases and their associated learning objectives. Using this file, project staff and curricular design groups could scan the curriculum for redundancies and gaps and select appropriate cases to cover proposed learning objectives.

Problem or case selection was another major determinant of what students chose to learn. Specific cases raised specific learning issues. Even when students were clearly determining what they would study, they were strongly affected by the case itself and the way it was presented. We learned that certain cases worked better than others in influencing the agenda for independent study.

The case writer, working with the curricular design group and an educator, developed learning objectives for each case. These objectives existed primarily for use by the tutor and were generally not shared with the students until they had an opportunity to define their own learning objectives. The tutor, knowing the objectives, could monitor the group's independent study plan and seek to modify the plan when the student group drifted too far afield. This turned out rarely to be necessary; most groups were as anxious as the case writers to cover what the case was intended to teach. The objectives were usually given to the students at the end of the case. We hoped that students might make a special effort later in the curriculum to return to objectives not covered earlier.

Vertical integration of cases and objectives was an important mechanism to encourage coverage of the essential knowledge, attitudes, and skills in the curriculum. We came to view the educational process as an ascending spiral through the four years wherein students reconsidered learning objectives of earlier cases in greater depth as a result of later experiences. Clinical cases during the third and fourth years offered such opportunities for student-directed learning to fill in learning objectives.

The tutor's competence was a critical factor in assuring that students achieved the learning objectives. In addition to steering the learning agenda, the tutor was the major source of quality control. By asking questions such as "How does that work?" "Why does that happen?" and "Are you sure about that?" the tutor could assure that students acquired more than superficial understanding of important mechanisms and concepts. The tutor had to steer a careful path between being overcontrolling or too directive and too undemanding or laissez-faire. Our faculty training program initially sought to help tutors feel comfortable with their role, but later turned increasingly to the issue of assuring competence.

Required Teaching Materials

Good case materials were essential to the success of the curriculum. Consistency of approach across blocks and good quality control were important goals. The project staff quickly developed a generic design for use in cases, emphasizing an appropriate fit between the length and complexity of the case, the students' level of sophistication, and the amount of time available. We determined that each case needed a listing of expert resources, a faculty guide including a list of references, and learning objectives.

Case writers were often conflicted about whether a case based on a particular patient should be modified to make it better achieve the desired learning objectives. We urged case writers to stick with the truth and to provide sufficient detail to the cases to raise psychological and social issues in addition to biological issues. Using real cases helped students understand that "real" medicine could be messy, unclear, and multidimensional and that at the same time one could strive for scientific exactitude.

Student Evaluation

We believed that the evaluation methods used in the New Pathway project would be major determinants of what and how students studied and learned. For this reason, we gave them special attention. Grading was either pass–fail or honors–pass–fail, at the discretion of the curricular design group director. Over time, pass–fail became more prevalent. The standard evaluation for each block comprised two elements: tutor assessment and feedback, and summative evaluation in the middle and at the end of each block.

Feedback and evaluation were used to help teachers and students understand where they stood with respect to educational standards and to encourage students to self-evaluate their progress. Feedback was to be given at least twice during the course, based upon a set of process objectives given to both students and tutors. The tutor's evaluation constituted half of the final course grade.

The other half of the grade was based upon formal summative assessment. We encouraged faculty to try new methods of testing, particularly seeking to develop approaches that could test the acquisition of learning skills themselves. While essay questions remained a major evaluation method, many of the blocks began to experiment with an approach initiated at McMaster University. In this method, students were given a case, asked to define learning objectives, and then were allowed several hours for independent study. After this time, a faculty member conducted a half-hour oral examination to determine the student's study methods, understanding of key concepts, and fund of knowledge.

Conclusion

Providing students with an optimal learning experience requires attention to both content and process. Traditional medical school curriculums concentrate on allocating time to different disciplines or departments; neither content nor the educational process is considered by a single centralized body in reviews and decisions. In the New Pathway curriculum, the Harvard faculty started by identifying overall educational goals that gave attention to process as well as to content, to attitudes as well as to knowledge and skills. Thus planning for the curriculum could follow broad guidelines in selecting learning objectives and the methods by which students would learn.

With attitudes and process included as salient goals of a medical curriculum, planners are freed from the most disabling of educational planning assumptions—that students must learn all the current scientific and clinical content during medical school. Under this assumption, as knowledge and applications increase, students must either work harder and faster or omit learning objectives deemed necessary by the faculty. A faculty can free itself to achieve its educational objectives only when its goal is to assure that students learn how best to learn and develop and maintain attitudes of intellectual curiosity and a commitment to keeping up-to-date. This goal, which requires a different kind of education, was the one adopted by the New Pathway project.

5

Curriculum Design

Elizabeth G. Armstrong
with Ronald A. Arky, Susan D. Block,
Daniel D. Federman, Alice S.-H. Huang,
Patricia J. McArdle, and Gordon T. Moore

C. Roland Christensen, veteran case teacher and University Professor at the Harvard Graduate School of Business Administration, has compared leading a case method discussion to conducting an orchestra. The leader requests the strings to play a bit louder, and then subdues them to hear from the woodwind section—all the while keeping the whole group in time and tune. Diverse players blend their unique talents into a melodious whole. So too, the curriculum plan of the New Pathway in General Medical Education aims to blend and integrate learning in biomedical, psychosocial, and clinical science areas. Its design responds to the 1984 recommendation by the Association of American Medical Colleges that the emphasis on the information-intensive approach to medical education be shifted to accommodate the acquisition and development of skills, values, and attitudes by weaving these themes into a kind of symphony, played over the four years of medical school.[1]

This chapter describes the specific content and organization of the original New Pathway curriculum and analyzes the methods used to integrate material within and across courses, to strike a balanced emphasis on process and content, and to harmonize self-directed learning with systematic presentation of the course material. In each interdisciplinary block, all three curricular themes are addressed in ways that help to blend the complex parts into a whole.

Design Overview

Two steps were essential to implement an interdisciplinary schedule by September 1985. The first step was to convene several interdisciplinary curricular design groups. Each was responsible for formulating objectives for a basic science block and articulating a set of teaching methods appropriate to accomplishing the objectives within the framework of the prototypical week (Figure 5.1). All the interdisciplinary basic science courses are designed and scheduled to fit this model while interweaving a full range of teaching modes. The second step was to determine the flow of the blocks and the number of weeks each would require (Figure 5.2). This was accomplished through discussions that frequently included strong faculty arguments for retaining a certain number of traditional lecture hours in the curriculum. The new curriculum integrates the lecture mode with case discussions in a way that we believe strengthens the learning potential of both.

Some of the tensions between lecture and case-discussion pedagogy in the faculty planning groups were resolved when instructors realized that reducing lecture time did not necessarily involve skimping on the content of any basic science. Despite a reduction in the number of

	Monday	**Tuesday**	**Wednesday**	**Thursday**	**Friday**
8:30 a.m.	Lecture	Lecture	Lecture	Lecture	Lecture
9:30 a.m.					
10:00 a.m.	Tutorial	Lab	Tutorial	Lab or Conference	Tutorial
12:00		Selective (2 hours)	Patient–Doctor (2 hours)		
5:00 p.m.					

Figure 5.1 Prototypical week for years I and II

	Human Biology	Patient–Doctor I	Selectives
Sept. Oct. Nov.	Human Body (8 weeks) Gross Anatomy Histology Radiology Cell Biology	Tutorial and clinical sessions alternate (34 sessions, 2 hours per week) First semester: Role of doctoring Patients' experience of illness Biopsychosocial model	One course in Social Medicine (2 hours per week) and One course in Biostatistics/ Epidemiology (2 hours per week) (Students select the semester in which they will take each course)
Nov. Dec. Jan.	Metabolism and Function of Human Organ Systems (11 weeks) Biochemistry Physiology Biophysics Molecular Biology		
Feb.	Pharmacology (4 weeks)	Second semester: Sensitive issues in history taking Basic interviewing skills	
Mar. Apr.	Genetics, Embryology, and Reproduction (6 weeks) Molecular & Human Genetics, Early Development, Morphogenesis & Reproduction		
Apr. May Jun.	Identity, Microbes, and Defense (10 weeks) Immunology Microbiology Pathology		

Figure 5.2 New Pathway curriculum, years I–IV

	Human Biology	Patient–Doctor II / Introduction to Clinical Medicine		Selectives
Sept.	Human Nervous System & Behavior (10 weeks)	14 1/2-day sessions Sept.–Dec.	History & physical exam skills	Psychopathology (3 hours per week)
Oct.	Neurology Psychiatry Neuroanatomy			
Nov.	Neurophysiology Neuropathophysiology			
Dec.	Medical Microbiology (7 days) Skin (1 week) — Focus on the patho-physiology of the major organ systems			
Jan.	Human Systems (9 weeks) Respiratory Cardiovascular Hematology			
Feb.	(15 weeks)	1 day/week for 8 weeks Feb.–Mar.	History & physical exam skills, including surgery and pediatrics	Preventive Medicine and Nutrition (2 hours per week)
Mar.	Endocrinology Reproduction Gastrointestinal Renal Musculoskeletal			
Apr.		2 days/week for 6 weeks Apr.–May		
May				

Figure 5.2 (continued)

Month	Patient–Doctor III			
Jul.	Introduction to the teaching hospital	(1 session)		
Aug.	HIV needle stick	(1 session)		
Sept.	Critical incident reports	(3 sessions)		3 critical incident reports, due in Sept., Dec., and Feb.
Oct.	Health finance policy	(3 sessions)		
	Risk management	(2 sessions)		
Nov.	Ethics	(8 sessions)		
	Social work rounds	(1 session)		
Dec.	Hospice/nursing home visits	(2 sessions)	37 tutorials and four large group meetings	
Jan.	Career choice	(2 sessions)		
	Death & dying	(3 sessions)		
Feb.	The ward team & students	(2 sessions)		Student assessment: 1 observed & videotaped clinical interview, Mar.
Mar.	Difficult patient	(3 sessions)		
	Cultural & ethnic issues	(4 sessions)		
Apr.	Clinical assessment	(1 session)		
May	Practicing prevention	(1 session)		
	Team projects	(4 sessions)		

Required Clerkships	Advanced Biomedical Science Program	Electives
Medicine (8 + 4 weeks) Ambulatory Care (8 weeks) Women & Children's Health (12 weeks) Surgery (8 weeks) Neurology (4 weeks) Psychiatry (4 weeks) Radiology (4 weeks)	Select 1 advanced biomedical science course (4 weeks)	Select clinical and other electives

Figure 5.2 (continued)

weeks allotted for discipline-based courses, the content of disciplines addressed in tutorials and independent study would make up that time overall in the interdisciplinary blocks. The change was in methodology, not in duration. In addition, the new courses permitted disciplines to work synergistically, as opposed to competing for time with other basic science courses. In the previous curriculum students had often had to assimilate unrelated content from many disciplines simultaneously. In the new system they could absorb various disciplines in an interrelated block.

The planners of each block interpreted the prototypical week slightly differently. The anatomists who designed the Human Body block adopted the most radical departure from traditional scheduling. In this block there are on average only three lectures per week, with daily one-hour tutorials and daily laboratories. Genetics, Embryology, and Reproduction combines three ninety-minute tutorials per week with one or two lectures per day and two clinics per week. The Human Nervous System and Behavior block follows the schedule of the prototypical week precisely. The flexibility of the prototype concept permits creative interpretations. Individual course directors have been able to mix and match strategies within the morning time frame. This design has increased faculty awareness of the need to include a variety of teaching modes in each block of time to encourage students to pay attention, become involved, and—most important—retain what they learn.

Courses

The following descriptions of individual courses further illustrate our design approach.

The Human Body (Year I)

This eight-week intensive introduction to basic anatomy and histology is centered on learning about the structure of biological systems from molecules to organisms. It is taught using problem-solving, case-based methods in small tutorial discussion sessions and laboratories. Medical cases guide and define learning agendas set by students as a group in their tutorials. Occasional lectures focus on general principles but do not systematically cover the course material. The laboratories offer hands-on experience in solving structural problems in cell biology, histology, gross anatomy, and radiology. The central focus of the course is to illustrate and integrate structural principles across all levels of magnification and to build a fundamental knowledge of the correlation between structure and function and of general systems rules.

Metabolism and Function of the Human Organ Systems (Year I)

This course consists of carefully linked parallel lectures in biochemistry and physiology, related both to each other and to the case of the week. For example, during the study of a case of diabetes mellitus, the physiology lectures address endocrine metabolism, and the biochemistry lectures focus on steroids and other modulators; and during tutorials on a case of chronic obstructive pulmonary disease, the physiology lectures present mechanisms of ventilation while the biochemistry ones present oxidative phosphorylation.

The course builds on students' basic knowledge of the structure and function of the human organ systems and aims to promote understanding of the interrelationships between structure and function at various levels of organization—from molecular to organismic. Selected topics in biochemistry, biophysics, physiology, and molecular biology are presented in a format that includes lectures, tutorials, conferences, laboratories, and computer-aided instruction. Emphasis is on the regulation of muscular, cardiovascular, gastrointestinal, respiratory, and renal function, the transport of water and solute, and on homeostasis and feedback regulation.

Principles of Pharmacology (Year I)

This four-week course on how drugs modify the body's mechanisms to alleviate or cure disease builds on the regulatory, physiological, and biochemical mechanisms of the human body studied in the first semester. Its primary objective is to communicate the action of the major classes of drugs and the principles underlying the formulation and evaluation of appropriate pharmacotherapeutic strategies.

Genetics, Embryology, and Reproduction (Year I)

This course focuses on fundamental aspects of human genetics, reproduction, early development, and morphogenesis. It addresses both classical and molecular genetics, with particular application to human biology and medicine. Laws that govern inheritance and variation among individuals and populations are considered, with special attention to the molecular aspects of inheritance, mutation, and gene control. New molecular, cellular, and cytogenic approaches are emphasized, with reference to human gene systems and inherited disease whenever possible. The endocrine events of puberty, the hormonal basis of human sexuality, and the control of gametogenesis are discussed. Lectures on early human development and the morphogenesis of selected organ systems are combined with tutorials, conferences, videotapes, or movies on other organ systems. All approaches are designed to help students visualize the developing organism in three dimensions. Major concepts of experimental embryology are introduced to assist the students in learning to think about developmental mechanisms.

Identity, Microbes, and Defense (Year I)

This is an interdisciplinary course that was extended to the entire first-year class in the spring of 1988, replacing separate courses in immunology, general pathology, and basic microbiology. The course emphasizes concepts basic to understanding the immune system, as well as the principles of microbial structure, metabolism, pathogenicity, and replication. It also explores the basic concepts of pathology, including injury, inflammation, hemostasis, atherosclerosis, and neoplasia.

Human Nervous System and Behavior (Year II)

This introductory course integrates the disciplines of anatomy, physiology, pharmacology, pathology, psychology, neurology, and psychiatry in the study of the functioning and malfunctioning of the nervous system. One clinical case per week introduces a wide range of issues by portraying patients whose symptoms require students to explore various areas of content. Topics covered by the cases include the general organization of the brain and spinal cord, localization of function, nerve impulse conduction, synaptic transmission, depression, addiction, personality structure, panic and anxiety, control of movement, sensory systems, psychosis, neuronal death and degeneration, cognitive function, and control of excitability in neuronal circuits.

A major activity in this course is independent study of topics identified as central learning issues in the clinical cases. After tutorial discussion, students broaden and deepen their knowledge alone or in study groups. Lectures help them to organize complex bodies of material, provide up-to-date information not readily available in textbooks, and consolidate material already studied. The laboratories, which have also been redesigned to offer more student-directed experiences, provide for the study of fixed tissues, radiological and scanning technology, and methods of electrical stimulation and recording. Short laboratory cases (one to three paragraphs) give students the human context for the pathology they are analyzing.

Human Systems (Year II)

This second-year block spanning twenty-six weeks focuses on the pathophysiology of the major organ systems and serves as a bridge to the clinical application of principles of basic science and physiology learned in previous courses. Units in the course include the respiratory, cardiovascular, endocrine, reproductive, renal, gastrointestinal, musculoskeletal, and hematologic systems. In addition, there are preliminary units on medical microbiology/infectious diseases and skin. Pathology, radiology, and pharmacology are integrated throughout the units. Clinical emphasis is increased, and cases challenge the students' problem-solving ability by incorporating diseases that affect multiple organ systems.

Patient–Doctor

Of all the courses developed for the new curriculum, this one underwent the greatest evolution from the time it was conceived for the pilot group (first two years) to its implementation for the entire class.

The patient–doctor relationship underlies all clinical practice, and the quality of the relationship has been shown to affect many factors, including health outcomes, patient satisfaction, and adherence to medical advice.[2] The need of physicians to improve their humanistic and interpersonal qualities is widely acknowledged.[3] Life-style-related diseases such as lung cancer, AIDS, and coronary artery disease have come to be major determinants of morbidity and mortality.[4] Social forces—poverty, lack of education, cultural differences—significantly influence the nature and experience of disease and illness.[5] Patients, clinicians, and scientists are increasingly recognizing the nature and extent of interactions between mind and body and their impact on how illness is experienced.[6] Ethical issues such as patient autonomy, decision-making about treatment, and balancing social and individual needs and resources are assuming increasing importance.

Yet there has been little focused and systematic teaching and learning during medical school about these fundamental issues and their implications for the patient–doctor relationship. Traditional medical school curriculums teach history-taking, obtaining the details of the patient's medical history, with relatively little attention to the interpersonal aspects of the interviewing process, such as ascertaining the patient's perspective on the illness and understanding the patient's social context and its meanings in relation to the illness. In general, students are not taught skills in patient education and counseling. Nor do they learn how to detect significant psychological disturbance and psychiatric illness in patients seen in medical settings. In fact, a dominant influence on students' styles of relating to patients is the attitudes of house officers, whose skills at relating to patients' psychosocial concerns and problems are often at their nadir and who often provide negative role models.[7] The longitudinal course on the patient–doctor relationship grew out of these concerns and values.

The experiment (years I–IV). Our approach to teaching and learning in this course was guided by an understanding that students enter medical school as adults, with a reservoir of experience and knowledge as well as a set of values that need to be respected, explored, and integrated into a highly personal style of approaching patients and doctoring. The educational process should provide opportunities for students to consider their own experiences and attitudes and should foster the development of an orientation towards self-reflection. Thus, stimulating students to be curious about the broadest aspects of their own patients became a central goal. Students began seeing patients during the first week of medical school and were encouraged to think, question, and explore their patients' experiences through group discussion, consultation, and reading.

In gathering a faculty, we sought to provide role models of effective interpersonal interactions with patients, of interdisciplinary respect and collaboration, and of respectful and reciprocal relationships as highly effective ways of encouraging students to develop these attitudes and skills. We hoped the relationship between teachers and students would mirror the qualities of empathy, respect, honesty, and reciprocity that should be present in physician relationships with patients. We exposed students to social and behavioral science concepts in the context of their efforts to understand clinical problems in order to demonstrate the utility and contribution of these domains to clinical medicine and to reinforce their attention to these issues.

The Patient–Doctor course began in the fall of 1985 with idealistic and optimistic goals, an ambitious course plan, complex logistics, both passionate and anxious teachers, and the students uncertain, excited, and ambivalent about the course material and methods.

Faculty and students found the course both intensely involving and overwhelming in its demands. Each preceptor group rapidly developed a sense of identity and an individualized approach to the course structure and material. A central tension in all the groups related to the question of how important it was to know the social/behavioral science material. The discussion and introspection about this question was itself a critical part of the course and encouraged each student to develop a personalized answer.

This conflict led the course organizers to articulate the course objectives more clearly and parsimoniously, to reduce and refine the readings, and to be more realistic about student involvement with patients. It also resulted in the deletion of expert-led colloquiums and in increased autonomy for the small groups in deciding what and how much to read, how closely to adhere to the course objectives, and how specifically to focus on the cases.

The second iteration of the course included a stronger emphasis on problem-solving with respect to the cases and encouraged students to take more responsibility for setting the learning agenda. Less material was covered in more depth.

An issue that has not been wholly resolved is the role of experts in social science, psychiatry, health promotion/disease prevention, clinical epidemiology, and medical humanities in relation to the role of clinicians. Achieving a reasonable balance between clinical and specialist orientations has proved difficult. In general, students responded more poorly to presentations of social science *qua* social science and were more open to social science concepts taught in the context of understanding patients. Basing social science teaching and learning solely on clinical cases, however, limited the depth of discussion and made it more difficult to address social and economic issues, which were not easy to discuss in the context of particular cases. Further, the clinicians tended to feel more comfortable when focusing discussion around individual patient issues and less competent and comfortable when opening up discussion to include more social, ethical, and economic issues.

The objective of having students follow a panel of patients throughout the course had to be modified. Instead, students followed one or two patients, often seeing them at home or when they were in the hospital, but not becoming care providers in the way originally envisioned. Nonetheless, several students became very involved with patients. The home visit, in particular, was a powerful experience in several instances and resulted in enduring attachments. One of the students, for example, followed his home-visit patient in the hospital during her terminal admission, went with the attending physician (his preceptor) and another student to her wake and funeral, and carried out a bereavement visit with the family several weeks later.

The current course (years I–III). The course is introduced in the first week of medical school and continues through the next three years. It is designed to promote professionalism and to integrate the basic and clinical sciences with the behavioral and social sciences.

In Patient–Doctor I, students learn firsthand from patients about the impact of illness and what patients expect from their physicians; they work closely with faculty to learn the fundamental skills of communicating and interviewing. Clinical sessions alternate with tutorial sessions and highlight clinical issues, including death and dying, AIDS, and approaches to the adolescent and to the difficult elderly patient. The impact of broad social issues on the care of the patient is introduced with discussions that center on gender, ethnicity, and culture; prevention and health promotion are integrated with discussions of respiratory illness or alcoholism. Selected literature from the social and behavioral sciences helps extend the students' understanding of attitudes, beliefs, and expectations that are brought to the clinical encounter by both patients and doctors.

Patient–Doctor II is designed to help students master the basic skills needed to perform a thorough physical and neurological examination. Almost all of the instruction, provided by a mixture of generalists and specialists, is hospital-based and continues throughout the academic year. Efforts are made to assure a close student–faculty relationship; ideally, faculty who have had contact with a student during the first year will retain some contact during the second. The teaching of specific skills in physical examination occurs simultaneously with instruction in related areas of pathophysiology. Thus, the essentials of the examination of the lungs and heart are presented at the same time students are concerned with problem-based cases in pulmonary and cardiovascular pathophysiology. The neurological examination and related interviewing skills are presented concurrently with student involvement in the neuroscience and introductory psychiatry courses.

During the year, at each of the eight hospital sites, the faculty coordinator leads discussions on ethical, social, economic, and other environmental issues that affect the patient–doctor relationship. These discussions are extensions and amplifications of related issues introduced in Patient–Doctor I. To facilitate the process and better utilize limited resources, specific sessions, such as those on pelvic and rectal examinations, are presented at the medical school instead of at the hospital sites. At least once during the year each student conducts a patient interview that is videotaped. The tapes provide resources for feedback by faculty on the student's performance and also afford measurable evidence of the student's progress in mastering interviewing skills.

Patient–Doctor III builds upon the first two years of the sequence and centers on discussions of the patients cared for during the students' clerkships. The close contact with patients during clerkships provides students with their richest and often most problematic experiences, but the hospital or ward environment affords limited opportunity to explore these issues with patients or family, faculty, and one another, and virtually no opportunities to read in disciplines related to medicine that would broaden understanding of these issues. For these reasons, Patient–Doctor III sessions are held weekly throughout the academic year, and the composition of tutorial groups resembles that of Patient–Doctor I; in some instances the students and faculty are the same.

Patient–Doctor III addresses all the crucial issues encountered by physicians in their professional activities. For example, students and faculty analyze the personal and ethical implications of commonly encountered clinical dilemmas, such as informed consent or defining the appropriate care for terminally ill patients. They discuss difficult patients—the chronically ill, the dying, those dealing with chronic pain or substance abuse—to improve their understanding of these problems, especially from the patient's perspective. Also explored are issues of health-care finance, risk management, and biases with regard to cultural, gender, or ethnicity differences.

Disease prevention, health promotion, nonconventional alternative treatment methods, and the range of career choices in medicine and the factors to be weighed in making such choices are also addressed in Patient–Doctor III. Students are encouraged to pursue in depth areas of special personal interest and to consider community-based service as group projects. From these discussions, their personal experiences, and the observations of peers, faculty, and nurses, students gain insight into their own attitudes of empathy, compassion, and understanding and recognize desirable and undesirable patterns. On three occasions during the academic year, the students formally relate these experiences in "critical incident" papers that serve as bases for both self- and group evaluation. Through these intimate interactions with peers and a supportive faculty, the concepts of professionalism are fostered and enhanced.

Issues in the Transition to the New Pathway Clinical Curriculum

Before the introduction of the New Pathway, the clerkships were organized in a traditional manner. Each specialty of medicine was offered in more than one of the teaching general hospitals, with each site planning its own content and teaching approaches. The New Pathway project established a single overall planning committee responsible for the twenty-three months of the students' third and fourth years. This group, working to achieve continuity with the curricular design groups for the first two years, was essentially the curricular design group for the third and fourth years.

The planning committee was responsible for rethinking the clerkships, planning their interrelationships, and attending to advanced basic science and advanced clinical electives. The result was an unfettered examination of and reflection on the knowledge, skills, and attitudes to be shared by all students. Once this work had been completed, committees were appointed for each of the major clinical disciplines. Membership was drawn from multiple sites and included basic science and extradisciplinary faculty. The goal of this organization was to ensure a cross-fertilization that is rare in the planning of specific clerkships. Working from agreed-upon objectives in the domains of knowledge, skills, and attitudes, each disciplinary committee was asked to define similar expectations for its own area.

The most radical change in the clinical years was not the revision of existing clerkships but the development of several new ones, including a two-month ambulatory care clerkship. This clerkship was created because planners doubted that the standard, teaching-hospital-based clerkships could be sufficiently modified to develop comprehensive and integrated presentation of ambulatory experience from diverse disciplines. The new clerkship includes medicine, pediatrics, and dermatology at clinical sites in the teaching hospitals, at the Harvard Community Health Plan, and in several outreach clinics affiliated with the teaching hospitals. Approximately half the time in this clerkship is dedicated to formal presentation and interdisciplinary problem-based discussions of chief complaints and problems that rarely present in the teaching hospitals. There is continuing discussion about whether this clerkship should focus on primary care or on the pathophysiology and therapy of the more complicated disorders for which hospitalization is either no longer used or is greatly abbreviated.

Another new clerkship combines women's and children's health. This three-month experience replaces two separate one-month clerkships in obstetrics-gynecology and pediatrics. It lengthens the inpatient experience in each discipline, adds an introductory week in which senior faculty present the special features of history-taking and physical examination of each discipline, and creates a mid-clerkship week of discussions about social and public health aspects of the two disciplines.

Changes in existing clerkships fell along a gradient ranging from creation of a teaching service for students separate from that for interns and residents in neurology to the addition of weekly conferences with a faculty member and one or two students in medicine. All the clerkships designed for the New Pathway placed greater emphasis on student-directed teaching and on contact with senior members of the faculty. The objectives of each clerkship were more clearly defined, with a core curriculum composed of clinical conditions each student must encounter during medical school. This approach is, of course, in use in many other schools and cannot be considered an innovation of the New Pathway project.

A seemingly minor change in the medicine clerkship has proved very successful. The former three-month experience, based on an ethos in which the student became "just like an intern," produced too much fatigue and pressure. The clerkship was broken into a two-month segment and an advanced one-month portion in which students could apply their learning from their surgery, ambulatory care, and women's and children's health clerkships and thus play a more sophisticated role but with less pressure.

The establishment of an overall committee under which each clerkship committee works has enabled us to specify interconnections, assign the presentation of specific topics, and ensure a comprehensive experience not available under the previous independent, segmented approach. The specification of a faculty tutor and the reexamination of overall content have led to changes in about 50 to 60 percent of the clinical curriculum.

Return to Basic Science in the Clinical Years

In another departure from the traditional curriculum, Harvard's New Pathway planners hoped to emphasize the "interweaving of clinical and basic science elements throughout the curriculum." This decision grew from the recurrent observation, articulated by Hilliard Jason, that "medical students think basic science is largely irrelevant to their real work and . . . have subsequently done little if anything, to bolster or reinforce either their store of basic science knowledge or their familiarity with basic science methodology."[8] The Harvard faculty reasoned that providing a clinical context for basic science learning and returning to explore basic science principles in the later years of the curriculum might assist students in applying the sciences to both clinical and investigative work during their careers.

The New Pathway planners identified two educational approaches for returning to basic sciences in the clinical years. First, they planned that students spend at least eight weeks on courses selected from a menu of clinically relevant basic science options. Second, reasoning that part of the general education of medical students should be concerned with understanding the investigative process, they required that each student undertake a thesis or project of at least two months' duration.

Advanced Basic Science Courses

At the time the faculty planners were wondering how to reintroduce basic science during the clinical years, the 1984 report of the Association of American Medical Colleges strongly recommended a return to basic science to enhance students' ability to utilize scientific principles and concepts in clinical problem-solving.[9] In 1984–85 only 13 percent of medical schools surveyed by Lila Croen and colleagues required students to return to a focus on basic sciences during their clinical years.[10] This study and experience at McGill University[11] suggested that designing such a learning experience would not be easy, since students wanted courses that were more clinical, and their achievement of scientific objectives declined as their focus became more clinical. Moreover, no studies documented that such courses enhanced students' use of basic science information in clinical practice.

The New Pathway planning group created two options for fourth-year students: at least eight weeks of signature courses, planned and given by outstanding clinical investigators, and a research project; or research leading to an honors thesis. A faculty director was appointed to develop course options and to oversee the student projects or theses.

At first, few new courses were developed. Scheduling courses around the clinical rotations presented a difficulty, since courses had to be given in two- or four-week blocks. Moreover, faculty were busy, accustomed to semester-long courses, and reluctant to give up a familiar format to develop new offerings; few were interested in designing courses for fourth-year students.

A few medical students attended graduate courses that were scheduled late in the day. Most students took existing courses in infectious diseases or biostatistics to fulfill their advanced science requirements. Earlier attempts in one of these courses to involve students in primary research publications had resulted in low attendance and complaints by the students and had been dropped. The basic science faculty did not view any of the available elective menu as meeting the definition of advanced science. Despite these initial problems, several interesting courses specially designed for the third group of students were developed for the 1989–90 academic year; these included molecular pharmacology, a course on mechanisms of disease, and a basic science course on neurosurgery. However, experience with these has been too brief to permit conclusions about the degree of their success.

The return to basic science lost considerable ground in the second and third years of the new program. In the first year the basic science reprise included both advanced science courses and an independent project for New Pathway students. During the second year the Curriculum Committee, in response to heavy lobbying from students, changed the requirement to either advanced science courses or an independent project, the so-called either/or requirement. In the third year, faced with too few advanced science courses to meet the demand, the faculty removed the requirement altogether. However, the either/or requirement was reinstated for the class of 1992.

These initial experiences afford several lessons. First, most medical students are resistant to taking basic science courses designed for graduate students. Drosophila genetics failed to attract medical students, no matter how well the course was taught. Special courses offered by clinicians with an appreciation of basic science seem to be far more attractive. Second, given the time constraints created by clinical rotations, faculty must attempt to develop new course formats and venues, such as one-month summer courses in places like Woods Hole where students could pursue complete involvement in one interest. Third, Dean's Office leadership and additional resources are needed to induce faculty to develop such courses and undergo training to teach them in a way that will be exciting to students fulfilling the requirement.

Student Thesis or Project

Although most Harvard faculty had long felt that all students should have an understanding and direct experience of the research method, only a small minority of medical school graduates had elected to prepare an honors thesis. The New Pathway planners envisioned that all students should undertake some type of investigative work as a prerequisite to graduation. Discussion with other schools that required a senior thesis suggested significant concerns. Students could be forced into projects in which they had little interest and end up doing trivial work. Such a required experience might cause exactly the opposite of the desired effect and actually reduce students' interest in and respect for the investigative process. Clearly, some students were already committed to the role of investigator and were fully prepared to undertake a major piece of research. Others, contemplating predominantly clinical careers, were unwilling to spend considerable time on a meaningful research project. Nevertheless, the planning group believed that these students, as well as those with a stronger basic science interest, should understand something about the nature of scientific investigation and acquire some of the skills of asking good questions and figuring out how to answer them.

The final design incorporated alternative ways to learn about research methods. Students could spend at least four to six months defining and carrying out a research project leading to a full thesis; they could participate in a more limited investigative exercise involving at least eight weeks of full-time work directly supervised by a faculty member; or they could prepare what was in effect a grant application in a subject of their interest, identifying an important and researchable question or hypothesis and pursuing the issue and its literature at great depth, but without doing the actual research. The result would be an extensive paper containing a statement of the purpose of the proposed study, a thorough review of the relevant literature, a description of the project's uniqueness and importance, a proposed research design, and descriptions of research methods and analytic methodologies. Students would critique one another's proposals under faculty guidance. The final product was intended to foster an understanding of the rules of evidence and the development of skills in communicating and presenting a line of argument in a persuasive manner. Students were expected to identify their approach to the thesis or project by the end of the second year and to select a faculty adviser during their third year.

The independent project, with its clearly stated expectations, enjoyed considerable success. Most students who undertook this requirement spent more than the minimum two months on their projects, and many chose topics in clinical and social sciences as well as basic sciences. None elected to do purely library research or to write a grant proposal. Each student presented an initial proposal for independent work, encompassing a hypothesis, background materials, methods to test the hypothesis, and methods to evaluate the results obtained.

Of the twenty-three students in the first New Pathway group, twelve fulfilled the project requirement by the expected graduation date. Almost all of them viewed the two-month exercise as a good one. One went on to do honors. One attempted to do laboratory research within the two months, met with equivocal results, but still felt that the experience was valuable. The remaining eleven students took more than four years to graduate, and almost all did more extensive research. Three obtained master's degrees, and another three entered the M.D.-Ph.D. program. One student spent a year doing research at the National Institutes of Health. This first New Pathway volunteer group appeared to be strongly motivated toward an academic/scientific career in medicine.

The second cohort of students had the option either to do an independent project or to take advanced science courses. Twenty-five percent chose to do the independent project, a proportion similar to that undertaking theses in the usual medical school class; thus it appeared that few students would volunteer for the experience if options other than the independent project were available. Some students, however, found the research so exhilarating that they exhorted their peers to take advantage of the opportunity for independent work. The success of such independent projects depends upon notifying students early about the option, helping them find suitable preceptors, and educating the preceptors about their responsibilities. A single central office with an updated roster of faculty and projects has been developed to facilitate the process and improve its quality.

Despite all the difficulties, we remain convinced that returning to basic science is an essential goal for the clinical curriculum. Investigation suggests that the most commonly employed forms of clinical reasoning and basic science thinking are largely separate cognitive domains, and that there may be a special role for basic science in providing "a basis for establishing and assessing coherence in the explanation of biomedical phenomena." In this model, science "provides the principles that make it possible to organize observations that defy ready clinical classification and analysis."[12] If this is the case, returning to basic science in the clinical years may be the way to assure that students learn how to link diagnostic reasoning and scientific principles and concepts when they most need it—when approaching unclear and uncertain clinical phenomena. In this model, basic science should be reviewed as students struggle to understand why and how clinical problems work.

The project or thesis appeared to be a successful mechanism for requiring students to learn how investigators ask good questions and proceed to solve them. The experiences were almost universally positive, and faculty generally applauded the depth and relative sophistication of the students' work.

Neither aspect of the return to science in the fourth year may be necessary for students to be effective in clinical decision-making. Nevertheless, these experiences have both theoretical and practical benefits in providing a foundation for remaining literate in medicine as our understanding of the mechanisms of health and illness evolves. By indicating that science is the tool that allows a clinician to answer the question "why," these courses both provide a foundation and reveal a method for keeping up-to-date and adapting and molding one's knowledge and skill over time.

Integration within and across Courses

According to Philip Leder, course director of the Genetics, Embryology, and Reproduction block, the objective of the New Pathway program to provide an integrating experience among the many medical disciplines has been met. Dr. Leder describes his own work planning this new curriculum as an attempt to meet a challenge from students and faculty to show why genetics should be integrated with embryology and reproductive physiology. His response has been to prove that genetics can be taught along with virtually any medical subject because it touches every aspect of human development. Reproductive biology also turns out to be a good fit with genetics because, as Leder explains, "much of what we have learned about reproductive biology follows from genetic disorders that have knocked out one or another function necessary for sexual maturation or development." The planning and design challenges in this course were to bring the distinct subjects of genetics, embryology, and reproduction together in a synergistic way and to find clinical examples with relevance to the three disciplines. Challenges like this are basic to the intention, design, and use of all our teaching cases.

Interdisciplinary integration has been relatively easy to achieve because we use "real life" medical cases, and the disciplines do converge in the practice of real medicine. The cases are drawn from actual medical records (disguised for confidentiality or obtained with a legal release), and efforts are made whenever possible to enliven each case with photographs, videotapes, epilogues from doctors and patients, relevant laboratory data, X-ray films, and ultrasound imaging. Occasionally the actual patient in the case is able to visit the class to be interviewed or to take part in a clinical presentation. We have also attempted to incorporate the psychosocial elements in the understanding of the patient's illness. Accordingly, the tutorial discussions in which the students gather to problem-solve and build new knowledge around a complex medical problem are broad-ranging.

Manfred Karnovsky, one of the designers of Metabolism and Function of the Human Organ Systems, compares the parallel lectures in biochemistry and physiology to the uprights of a ladder, and the case tutorials to its rungs: they "not only hold the structure together but provide the footholds for the user, who may thus ascend to greater heights." After the first three months of the block the "uprights" begin to draw closer to each other as the lectures cover ever more closely related phenomena.

Robert B. Colvin, the director of Identity, Microbes, and Defense, a ten-week course at the end of the first year, likens the integration of general pathology, immunology, and microbiology to the progressive interweaving of three strands of a rope to increase its strength. Dr. Colvin constantly emphasizes the interrelatedness of the three subject areas in the real-life practice of medicine. Because he believes that physicians must bring knowledge of many disciplines to bear on a patient's problem, he supports the idea that the habit of integrating knowledge should begin in the first year of medical school.

Early each academic year Colvin, the course codirectors, and their curriculum coordinator begin planning for the spring course. They consider the essential concepts to be presented, the logical progression through the material, and the best format for meeting the educational goals of the course. They emphasize basic disease mechanisms, integrative knowledge, certain practical laboratory skills, critical analysis, and independent study.

The central case for each week supports an analysis that dovetails with the content of lectures and laboratories. Time is allotted for three ninety-minute case-discussion tutorials per week. The director and codirectors, in consultation with others in their departments, then plan the lectures (approximately one per day), laboratory exercises, and conferences to fill the rest of the morning hours. Colvin reviews and approves the total plan but rarely interferes with decisions of the codirectors.

In the course guide, the tutorials are described as the backbone of the course.[13] All other exercises are limbs (some with a lot of muscle) that gain leverage and form from the cases. Course codirectors write the cases in conjunction with several other faculty members. Each case is then scrutinized by a case review group that includes an experienced tutor, several students who have previously taken the course, and the curriculum coordinator. New cases are introduced each year, and old cases are reviewed and revised on the basis of formal feedback from tutors and students. In the future, tutorial groups may be able to choose the cases they wish to study from a bank of approved cases on various topics.

The cases are carefully chosen and written to avoid random summary and to serve as vehicles for meaningful learning. Faculty tend to eschew the minimalist approach to case writing. They include references, objectives, vocabulary lists, names of faculty members willing to serve as "expert resources," and a tutor guide. Each basic case narrative runs from ten to twelve pages in length. Students receive modular units of one or two case pages at a time as they work their way through the events of the case in chronological order with their tutors. Faculty-designed objectives or guiding questions are not given out until approximately halfway through the study of the case to allow students to think broadly at first and to set their own learning agendas. Students are expected to integrate their knowledge and understanding of each new subject area as it emerges from the analysis of the cases. Thus, for example, by the end of the course, principles of pathology, immunology, and microbiology are brought to bear on the study of an AIDS case.

To support continuity over the four years while minimizing redundancy and overlap, we have installed a customized computer-based Curriculum Index. From this database system faculty can obtain a list of courses in which a particular topic is addressed, together with the teaching material used. Curriculum planners can use it to review potential avenues for updating existing objectives, revising cases, and improving lectures or other teaching strategies. The Curriculum Index has already helped us to define our content in medical ethics, preventive medicine, and AIDS and to weave these topics into the fabric of existing interdisciplinary courses at increasingly sophisticated levels without threatening their integrity.

The creation of an interdisciplinary curriculum both within and across blocks has had far-reaching effects on the faculty. Coming together with specialists from other disciplines to plan and teach these courses has offered unprecedented opportunities to maintain and strengthen fruitful collegial alliances. Some faculty report that their research and clinical practices have been influenced by this productive involvement in course planning and curriculum review.

The New Pathway program has also drawn far more faculty into the teaching effort than previously participated in the traditional lecture-based curriculum, which required planners to organize courses around lecturers' busy schedules. The new courses typically require about twenty tutors, twenty laboratory instructors, up to twenty conference leaders, and an appropriate set of lecturers who are asked to provide a series of presentations. Not all blocks have laboratories and conferences. With the new set of teaching roles and the careful intercalation of teaching strategies, up to 100 faculty members may work together in a given course. All require, and receive, information about the multiple components of the course.

The Human Body block differs from all others in its record of recruiting faculty from the former Department of Anatomy and Cellular Biology to serve as tutors, laboratory instructors, and lecturers. Daniel A. Goodenough, the course director, comments:

> The new curriculum requires the students to learn to use teamwork; it is thus critical for the faculty to teach with teamwork. The development of a single course that integrates both the microscopic and gross anatomy has had the delightful consequence that a departmental group spirit has emerged. All faculty in the department are required to teach the same material, all must attend the laboratories, all have equivalent tutorial groups, and all experience the same number of teaching hours, from Assistant to Full Professor. Since the course is taught during an intense eight-week period, the faculty all simultaneously turn their attention to the teaching at the same time, find themselves in the teaching spaces together, and are thus able to join in collegial interactions around teaching excitement and prob-

lems. The result is a common collective energy, a sense of teamwork, which builds upon itself as the course progresses, and substantively helps in the maintenance of high levels of enthusiasm and commitment.

Shared Emphasis on Process and Content

Early in the New Pathway curriculum planning, discussions of the traditional four-year curriculum often referred to the need to "prune" its highly factual content. The popularity of this term reflected a parallel realization that methods of teaching and learning also required careful examination. The curriculum planners wanted not simply to reduce factual content; they wanted to improve student retention and grasp. In their deliberations about adult learning they included discussions of a range of teaching styles enlightened by modern cognitive psychology and agreed that teaching methodologies would have to be designed and implemented to support self-directed learning. Moreover, teachers would model behaviors that students could emulate in their own interactional styles with patients. Teaching took on a whole new perspective. Content shared the stage with process.

All the descriptions of the new interdisciplinary courses emphasize mechanisms and principles over simple fact. According to Daniel Goodenough,

> Rather than try to expose the students to as much content material as possible in the brief time allowed, "covering" all the "important" information in a coruscation of faculty recitation, an effort has been made to focus on structural principles and concepts, and to trust the students to commit themselves as adult learners to the process of studying biological structure all their professional lives, continuously revisiting the skills obtained in our brief course as they encounter structural problems in their own personal career paths.
>
> Thus, a single example of how a molecule is combined to make macromolecules, cells, tissues, organs, and organisms is selected, in this case collagen, and the application of these rules to many other countless molecules, normally "covered," is left for the student to uncover as the fabric of basic science unfolds driven by each student's individual experience and curiosity. The students focus in detail on the principles of limb anatomy by studying one limb, not both, with the belief that the salient features of both limbs will be revisited in many different, relevant contexts. A particular case may focus on

one aspect of thoracic anatomy, leaving other details of the gross and microscopic structure of the chest to unfold during later experiences. Our teaching goals hold foremost that the student will appreciate the need to be able to think structurally, will have developed confidence that s/he can, with appropriate resources, clearly think through any structural problem, and will thus be trained as a lifelong student of structure, always aware that there must be continuous study and learning.

Evaluation

Donald E. Melnick, Director of the Division of Research and Development at the National Board of Medical Examiners, has recently criticized the current National Board of Medical Examiners examination for merely measuring knowledge of a dense conglomerate of facts without emphasizing the need for physicians to apply this information or to understand its interrelationships.[14]

As the New Pathway program has evolved, our course directors have come to the realization, along with the National Board of Medical Examiners, that their examinations should assess the degree to which students have integrated biomedical facts into a cohesive knowledge base and the degree to which the information is understood and transferable to new applications. Because evaluation instruments determine what students perceive as the real goals of any curriculum, our student assessments aim to reflect the shift in emphasis from rote recall of huge numbers of facts to application, analysis, and synthesis of a flexible knowledge base.

An example of one of the new examination formats, designed in the Identity, Microbes, and Defense course, is called the Quadruple Jump. Course planners strongly believe that examinations should have educational value in and of themselves and should be congruent with the stated interdisciplinary objectives of the course. Based on the Triple Jump, developed by Alexander Powles and colleagues at McMaster University,[15] this examination tests problem-solving skills, self-study, the ability to synthesize and apply concepts, and the demonstration of certain practical laboratory techniques.

Students are given a description of a case they have not previously seen. They immediately write a brief analysis of the case and a proposed study agenda on a carbon set and turn in one copy. In the ensuing hours the students pursue an in-depth study of the case, using any personal notes or library or computer resources available. They also perform a laboratory analysis of material from the case. On the following day each student takes an oral examination administered by a team drawn from the tutors, laboratory instructors, and course planners. During the first half of the examination the student presents an analysis of the case and what he or she has learned about it. The examiners follow up with questions, either probing related areas or leading the student into an extension of the analysis. The last few minutes are used to give the student immediate feedback.

Students are enthusiastic about this method of examination. When it was used for the final examination of the entire class for the first time in June 1989, students gave it a 1.6 rating on a scale of 1 to 5 (1 = highest). Comments included:

> "I didn't feel that I was just reciting. I had to think, which was fun. The examiners probed what I knew well, not threateningly."
>
> "I really enjoyed this well-written and well-executed test. I got to learn about a very important disease and apply my knowledge from many different areas of the block."
>
> "It was a great experience. The case was tough, but it brought out a lot of important issues."
>
> "This was a great idea. Although I was very nervous about the oral portion of the exam, I feel as if I learned a great deal, and I will never forget Hepatitis B infection."

This type of evaluation and those designed for the other interdisciplinary blocks focus on solving problems rather than on reciting facts and reflect the commitment to challenge students to think at a higher level in the cognitive domain. Course goals that call for equipping the student with the tools to obtain, assess, and utilize new information demand instruments of evaluation that measure objectives that are less readily observable and measurable than formerly.

The Tutorial

The cornerstone of the Human Body block is the tutorial group. Group work involves learning activities at many levels, including informational, conceptual, attitudinal, characterological, and interpersonal. This approach reflects the role modeling of character, commitment, ethics, and self-awareness, as well as an understanding of group process. These concepts are not simply discussed in the abstract in behavioral science courses.

The students begin with medical cases, with all their complexity, richness, and humanity. The experience is initially overwhelming. The students' first response is to rush to medical textbooks, to try to be a "doctor." But they realize rapidly that they must first learn some basics (what's inside the chest?).

The cases are studied in a small group (six to eight persons), which provides an environment of peers in which it is safe to admit ignorance. Because the faculty group leader also cannot know all there is to know about the case and does not control the agenda for the discussion, she or he must also admit ignorance, contributing to, role-modeling, the safety. The group must discuss and agree on goals and develop common meanings. This process allows students and teachers to define what they don't know and what they need to know. The group must prioritize these needs, set agendas, and explore study strategies. Differences arise immediately and must be negotiated; the necessity fosters appreciation of the richness offered by difference. This process of group formation is exquisitely complex and occurs at different rates for different groups.

The goal of any group session is not to arrive ignorant and to leave filled with knowledge. Rather, the goal is to arrive with the wealth of information already acquired in life, find the edge of both personal and general knowledge, then leave excited, motivated, directed, and responsible to the group. This is the frame of mind conducive to self-directed learning, stimulated by necessity, curiosity, and peer pressure.

The goal of the Human Body block planners is to create an environment in which students can succeed best through teamwork. They select cases with the potential to generate questions that go to the heart of the content of the course, questions that are straightforward to ask but require rigorous scientific inquiry and study to answer. For example, in a case involving chest pain, in which the patient experiences "shortness of breath," the questions arise: What could cause shortness of breath? How do we breathe? When we exhale, how come the air comes out of our lungs without our having to actively push it out? When we strain while lifting a weight, why does our breakfast stay in our stomachs? How do we blow up a balloon? The questions rapidly immerse the students in thick and complex textbooks of anatomy, physiology, and biochemistry. In their groups they must either build a collective raft of knowledge or flounder and sink in a sea of information.

Since the goals of the course include thinking about biological structure and function at all levels of magnification, it is necessary to help students construct a conceptual framework: a set of structural rules for living systems. So questions include: What is a system, and how do we see one? What are the boundaries of a system, and what are their properties? As students probe the boundaries of the cell, for example, they discover that cell membranes are continuous, semipermeable, asymmetric, heterogeneous, and dynamic, that they change shape by expansion and contraction from within. Functionally, boundaries are dialectical, providing both separation and connection, thus permitting differentiation. But these rules also apply to boundaries at larger levels of structure, such as skin and the lining of the intestines. And when the discussion really gets going, sometimes the group discovers that they themselves are a system, and that the group has boundaries with the same structural and functional rules. In these sessions, students might discover that their individual boundaries, which at first they might have thought to be their own skin, are in fact much more complex: our level of comfort is affected by how close someone sits to us, even without touching our skin. This realization leads to an understanding that our boundaries change depending on our context: we can stand very close to a stranger on a crowded elevator but not on an unpopulated beach. Boundaries are defined by contexts and goals. And, down the magnification ladder, is this true of cellular boundaries as well? Back up: what happens to our boundaries when we go to see the doctor?

Balancing Self-Directed Learning with Systematic Coverage

> Learning is self teaching . . . The Teacher's part, then, in the process of instruction is that of a guide, director or superintendent of the operations by which the pupil teaches himself.
>
> —Joseph Payne, *Lectures on the Science and Art of Education* (1883)

The idea that adult learners teach themselves is scarcely revolutionary. By incorporating this idea as its first principle, and augmenting it with an acknowledgment of the range of adult learning styles born of modern cognitive psychology, the New Pathway curriculum displays what might be considered its most characteristic quality, hybridization. As new musical styles build upon the old, our curriculum aims to innovate without sacrificing the best of the old, to stimulate individual initiative without inefficiency, and to balance the latest developments in medical science with the age-old values of healing. In every sense, our goals and the implementation of these goals are hybrids—with, we hope, the strength and adaptability that hybrids usually display.[16] The designers of the prototypical week (Figure 5.1) played an important role in creating the hybrid through their recognition of the need to maintain a variety of teaching modes. Lectures were retained but altered in format and frequency. Laboratories and conferences were interspersed in the tutorial sequence. Finally, designers required that all teaching strategies aim to become more student-directed and that the content addressed in each be carefully interrelated.

Our hybrid model differs from the traditional first- and second-year medical curriculum in having fewer contact hours and lectures per week and in balancing case discussions with lectures, laboratories, clinics, and conferences. Within the existing weekly schedule, lectures are presented as a multidisciplinary series whose theme relates to the teaching objectives of the week. All of the approaches combine to support student learning at a level that enhances the potential application of a broader knowledge base. From this perspective, the reduction of the number of lecture hours and the possible decrease of information conveyed in this format are compensated by gains in students' ability to solve problems and ask questions and in their motivation to seek out and develop answers.

Conclusions

Arthur Kaufman has suggested that problem-based learning can take root in an institution only if a broad spectrum of the faculty implements it.[17] The Harvard Medical School curriculum shift has accomplished just that. By creating a curriculum that promotes active learning and self-direction in harmony with a variety of other teaching modes, we have tapped large numbers of faculty as tutors, lecturers, laboratory leaders, conference leaders, and clinical clerkship instructors. Teaching has become the responsibility of many faculty in disparate areas as they work toward common goals—not only in interdisciplinary content areas but also in a shared commitment to helping students succeed as self-directed adult learners.

Having now developed our own network of faculty to design and implement a new curriculum that supports self-directed learning in a variety of teaching modes, we acknowledge the need for the same sort of continuing self-assessment that we expect of our students. Our perpetual question must be: How well does our curriculum support learning? As students, faculty, and society change, new technologies in teaching will also emerge. Discovering new content and new processes over the next decades will require us to apply all the problem-solving skills that we expect our students to acquire. For those of us who design, implement, and evaluate curriculums, each new iteration is a case in problem-based learning for us to analyze.

6

Faculty Development

LuAnn Wilkerson

Numerous studies of the adoption of curricular innovations suggest that the characteristics of the innovation itself, the organization, and the individual adopter interact to facilitate or subvert the process of change.[1] First, the likelihood that an individual will adopt an innovation, particularly one that will require new patterns of behavior, is increased when the innovation meets a perceived need and when utilization produces an individually rewarding outcome. Second, the individual must perceive the innovation as being compatible with personal values, beliefs, and behavioral skills. This criterion may be even more powerful a predictor than that of perceived need. Third, since the individual is a member of a complex social and professional system, having colleagues whom one respects support the innovation exerts a powerful influence on actual adoption. This chapter explores how an institutional commitment to faculty development and the evaluation of educational contributions were used to encourage the adoption of curricular change.

The chapter begins with the stories of two Harvard Medical School faculty members and their disparate journeys into the New Pathway project. These stories illustrate critical issues raised by a move into any new curriculum that demands new ways of thinking and acting as a teacher and highlight the central role played by individual faculty in determining the success of a new curriculum. The rest of the chapter describes the various actions taken in response to perceived faculty needs and suggests principles for designing faculty development and evaluation programs.

The Case of the Coerced Biologist

John was an Associate Professor of Anatomy and Cellular Biology with an active research program on the role of the cytoskeleton in reproduction and early development, using the sea urchin as a model system. As initial plans were being made in 1983 for the New Pathway course called the Human Body, which would combine what were traditionally two courses, histology and gross anatomy, John volunteered to remain with the existing histology course rather than tutor in the new curriculum. In 1985 he became codirector of the histology course and began to reorganize the lecture series, including developing several new lectures of his own. By the spring of 1987 he was extremely proud of the results of his efforts and glad that the school had maintained a two-track curriculum, since it offered him a chance to lead his own course.

When the members of his own department, enthusiastic about the New Pathway approach in the Human Body, started the movement that led to the adoption of a New Pathway curriculum for all incoming students in the fall of 1987 (see Chapter 10), John was not among their ranks. He was informed by his department head that his course in histology would no longer be a part of the medical student curriculum and he would have to become a tutor and laboratory instructor in the new course. His first reactions were anger and anxiety. He had worked extremely hard to design the histology course and spent hours planning his own lectures, preparing slides, and writing examination questions—when he could have been writing grants. Now, in spite of positive student ratings, his course was being abandoned.

His anxiety stemmed from several sources. First, as a cell biologist, he had found teaching histology something of a challenge, but he had enjoyed reconnecting with his earlier studies of cellular architecture. As a tutor in the Human Body, however, he would be expected to discuss material covering all aspects of histology and gross anatomy, to say nothing of the issues in clinical medicine raised by the inclusion of clinical cases. Then there were the laboratories. Histology laboratory was familiar ground, but he had never seen a cadaver, much less touched a scalpel to human skin. In previous years he had heard students deriding faculty who did not know the answers to their esoteric questions. How could he possibly master sufficient content between April and September to face a group of students who would quickly uncover his lack of expertise in the course content?

Although the idea of the problem-based tutorial was somewhat disturbing, he was attracted to the idea of working with a small group. He recalled that his best educational experience in college had been a small-group project in which the students "discovered" Greek. However, all of his previous teaching experience had been as a lecturer in the amphitheater or laboratory. If you knew your stuff cold, organized it clearly, wrote a complete handout, and threw in a little humor, you were bound to succeed. What would it take to be a successful tutor?

John had seen a demonstration tutorial in January 1987 at a faculty conference on problem-based learning. He and his colleagues from anatomy who had not yet been a part of the New Pathway program were persuaded that students were, just as they had suspected all along, interested only in learning to diagnose and treat symptoms, not in learning basic science. They could not imagine that taking away the handout, replacing well-organized lectures with chaotic discussion of clinical cases, and adding time for radiology conferences would lead to the learning of histology and gross anatomy. The demonstration tutorial by the second-year students in the Oliver Wendell Holmes Society had just proved them right! It was all too clinical. He did not know medicine, nor did he have time to learn it.

Then the Human Body course director had invited him to participate as a "student" in a practice tutorial using a case of X-ray crystallography. He had enjoyed trying to solve the puzzles but felt totally overwhelmed when he had to work them at the board in front of the group. Tutorial had to be a safe place if students were to expose their ignorance. But he wondered if students would really know what to learn if you did not tell them. What if no one said anything in tutorial, but all just looked to him for the answers, particularly clinical answers?

These questions and concerns continued to nag John as he entered the first tutorial in September 1987. He decided that the best way to begin was to be honest about not knowing exactly how to proceed and then to offer some structure within which the group might begin its work on the first case. At least then he could exert some measure of control over what he thought would otherwise be unproductive chaos. During that first week, the students tried hard to follow the structure that John had outlined, and in fact the tutorial worked better than he had thought it would at delving into basic science. As he was listening, he found it easy to remember students' names and to pick up interesting bits of information about them as individuals, about their previous experiences, and what they already knew about anatomy. However, by the fourth day, it was clear that there was some continuing discomfort with the tutorial process. Although the students all participated eagerly, far beyond his initial expectation, their discussion was wandering and unfocused.

At the end of the first week, John asked the students to evaluate the experience thus far. He began by stating his own continuing concern about not knowing enough to be helpful to them. After a long silence, Scott smiled, looked around at the other students in the group and offered a different version of the problem: "You see yourself as outside of the group and we see you as a member. Don't worry about what you should be doing. We can figure it out together."

With a sigh of relief, John sat back, and the students began to talk about their own anxieties in beginning medical school, finding themselves in a new type of learning experience, being afraid to be wrong, not knowing what to learn. Over the next few tutorials, they began to develop strategies for helping one another learn with John as an equal member of the group. Three years later, they still had an occasional reunion and laughed about those first halting steps together. John became an enthusiastic supporter of the student-directed, problem-based approach, a skilled and caring tutor, and a resource for new faculty just learning to tutor. After his third year as a tutor, the students and faculty honored his contributions to the New Pathway with an Excellence in Teaching award.

The Case of the Physician Who Loved to Teach

Joan volunteered early to be part of the planning group for the Patient–Doctor course, a new approach to teaching clinical skills that combined the power of a longitudinal relationship with a mentor and a problem-based tutorial approach to behavioral science learning. She was pleased that the new course would give primary care faculty a central role in the curriculum. She found several features of the Patient–Doctor course particularly attractive, since they seemed to correct problems that she had experienced in her own education and corresponded to her own professional values: a psychosocial orientation, early patient contact, an emphasis on eliciting the patient's perspective, continuity-of-care experience, and an opportunity for a longitudinal mentoring relationship.

Although her primary care practice was busy and most of her previous teaching experience was with residents, she was eager to move beyond the planning phase and to serve as a preceptor for the first cohort of students in the New Pathway project. Her division chief was supportive, although he expressed some concern about the potential loss of income to the faculty group practice as a result of a course that took three to four hours a week for a three-year period.

As a preceptor, Joan would share responsibility for leading a weekly problem-based tutorial with another internist and a psychiatrist or social scientist. In addition, she would supervise two of the six students in their learning of clinical skills. Initial plans called for this group of faculty and students to stay together over the entire course.

In the fall of 1985 the first students arrived. Joan's two preceptees were curious and eager to learn. The tutorial group seemed to function much like attending rounds. Someone would summarize the assigned paper case and then she would guide the discussion with a variety of pointed and provocative questions. She thought having the other faculty members present provided for multiple perspectives, although she had to admit that sharing leadership of the group was a little difficult.

During the first month of the course, I asked if I might observe the tutorial group. On the day I sat in, all four faculty members assigned to the team were present, and they were clearly having as much fun with the material as were the students. Afterward Joan and I talked about strategies for giving the students a larger role in setting the agenda for discussion and reducing faculty contributions without squelching faculty enthusiasm. After watching the students closely over the next several weeks, Joan discovered that tutorial discussion could be much more student-directed and that fewer questions were needed from her to keep the discussion going.

When her two preceptees finished the three-year Patient–Doctor sequence, Joan returned to the first-year curriculum as a member of the advisory group for the course. During the next year the original tutorial group continued to meet on a social basis to discuss career choice and internship applications. Joan loved the continuing contact with the students and felt that over time she had developed a particularly meaningful relationship with her two preceptees, both of whom were thinking seriously about primary care. Moreover, she felt that her own clinical practice had improved as a result of her continued reading and thinking about the issues raised in the course. In 1989 Joan became course director for Patient–Doctor I.

In spite of her contributions to the new curriculum as a tutor, preceptor, and course director, Joan did not expect any change in her academic status. Although she had recently written two chapters in an important textbook, participated in several clinical studies, cochaired a national educational meeting of and held offices in her professional specialty group, and served as associate director of the ambulatory component of the primary care residency training program in her department, she still held the rank of instructor with which she had begun at Harvard Medical School in 1977. Several years earlier she had decided to follow her own interests rather than be driven by the academic reward system. Consequently she had ceased to worry about how to devote more time to research and had become increasingly involved in student and resident teaching programs.

As a result of several circumstances, including the renewed emphasis on teaching created by the New Pathway project, a new set of criteria for promotion, the Teacher-Clinician track, was introduced in the spring of 1988. These criteria were parallel in structure to the existing criteria for advancement in basic research or clinical investigation, with no differentiation in title or appointment duration. Joan was the first junior faculty member promoted under the new criteria in the spring of 1989. In the spring of 1990 the graduating class named her "the best clinical teacher."

Faculty Development and Evaluation

Problem-based learning requires teachers to reexamine the relationship between what they do and what students learn, a task for which John was initially unwilling and unprepared. The old notion of learners as empty vessels just waiting to be filled by the teacher's expertise is no longer appropriate. Research in cognitive psychology, neurophysiology, and education has created a new, more active view of learning in which learners are not passive recipients of prepackaged knowledge but instead are actively working to construct meaning out of the experiences and educational tasks in which they are involved.[2] This new educational paradigm calls for new relationships between teachers and students, changes that lie at the heart of the New Pathway curriculum.[3] The role of the teacher is also altered.[4] Rather than organizing and transmitting information, the teacher guides and shapes the work of learning.[5] Like a coach, he or she is watching from the sidelines, encouraging and correcting while students run the plays. Few medical school faculty are prepared for these crucial roles.[6] This lack of preparation is not surprising; the intensity and duration of medical and doctoral-level training leave little time for study of the process of education, learning theory, and teaching strategies or for the evaluation of learning. As a result, faculty tend to teach in the same ways in which they were taught. Most are unaware of the differential impact of learning tasks on individual students, do not state expectations explicitly, are less than systematic in their evaluation practices, and equate teaching with lecturing. Like John, when faced with a curricular change that calls for new ways of behaving as an individual, faculty members often resist the unknown.[7]

In the New Pathway project, faculty like John and Joan were asked to take on several nontraditional teaching roles: as tutors in interdisciplinary student-directed, small-group discussion; as consultants to students who had already studied intensively in a particular area; as mentors with a longitudinal responsibility for the development of professional skills and attitudes; and as evaluators of both cognitive and affective learning. Even the role of the lecturer was different, with a responsibility not so much to transmit a plethora of facts as to provide an orienting framework or to explicate topics found confusing by students during tutorial discussion.

Because most of the New Pathway courses in the first two years are interdisciplinary, tutors experience some initial anxiety about their ability to listen critically or to guide discussion in the areas outside their expertise.[8] As a faculty becomes more specialized, finding teachers for any medical curriculum becomes more difficult. Although John did not have to devote more time to teaching as a result of the new curriculum, Joan's division chief warned her not to devote too much time to student education. A study of faculty time in tutoring at the University of New Mexico suggests that the total number of hours needed from an individual tutor is not necessarily greater than that needed by a lecturer in the traditional curriculum.[9] However, the distribution of that time between student contact and preparation is strikingly different. In the problem-based curriculum at the University of New Mexico, tutors spend 72 percent of their time with students and 28 percent in preparation, whereas faculty in the traditional curriculum spend 61 percent of their time in preparation.

In a 1987–88 survey of tutors in the eleven-week Metabolism and Function of the Human Organ Systems course, we found that, on average, each of the twenty tutors spent 38 hours in tutorial, 8 hours meeting individually with students, 13 hours in faculty development and case review, 31 hours in individual study, 8 hours attending course lectures, and 3 hours writing evaluations, for an average of 101 hours, or about two average work-weeks per year. The results of an identical survey in 1988–89 suggest that individual preparation and attendance at lectures dropped substantially during a tutor's second year of participation.

To place in perspective the figure of 101 hours for a new tutor, compare the estimate given by a previous course director of hours spent in preparing and giving a new lecture in the traditional curriculum: 1 hour in class, 1 hour after class in informal discussion, 40 hours preparing the handout, 4 hours for notes and slide preparation, 2 hours writing examination questions, 10 hours attending other course lectures, and 12 hours attending meetings of conference leaders on material related to the lecture, for a total of 70 hours. For a repeat lecture, the preparation time dropped considerably, to 3 to 8 hours. These numbers suggest that either curriculum demands a substantial commitment of time. At Harvard Medical School, where there was previously no requirement that every faculty member teach, participation is now distributed among many faculty members to keep the total number of hours low, with contributions as tutor, lecturer, or laboratory instructor limited to only one course and/or core clerkship. Schools with fewer faculty might involve faculty in multiple roles or multiple courses, with a concomitant increase in teaching time for individuals.

On the other hand, the Patient–Doctor course, with its weekly alternation between clinical skills sessions and tutorials throughout the year, is extremely faculty intensive. As a tutor and preceptor, Joan would be involved with students for two to three hours a week for thirty weeks during the year plus individual meetings, patient recruitment, and faculty development. Clearly, this contribution represents a substantial teaching commitment—on the order of 5 to 8 percent of an individual's total work effort over a year. The new clerkships, with their emphasis on more student–faculty contact, also require the involvement of more faculty or more time from those currently teaching.

Because the institution needed more time from its clinical faculty for these reforms, it had to devise ways of encouraging and rewarding previously underemphasized and unrewarded academic contributions to the first two years. At present, many of the tutors in both the basic science core courses and the Patient–Doctor course are physicians.

Addressing this issue was particularly urgent for the New Pathway project, since it would require the dedicated participation of faculty members in teaching outside their own disciplines. Interdisciplinary teaching activities must be documented in an effective and visible way for the faculty member's own department. Belief that the institution is genuinely committed to the recognition and reward of educational scholarship and the exemplary practice of teaching seems essential to the recruitment, training, and retention of faculty planners and teachers in the new curriculum.

Research has demonstrated that teachers can and do improve their performance, given appropriate opportunities for learning and a reward system that encourages participation in teaching.[10] However, the planners of the new curriculum believed that many faculty would be unable to fill their new roles effectively without careful preparation and expert assistance in reexamining their teaching assumptions and practices.

Initial Recommendations

In 1983, as initial planning of the new courses was getting underway, the New Pathway Steering Committee formed an Ad Hoc Committee for Faculty and Case Development to analyze the first steps necessary in implementing new course plans by the fall of 1985. This group realized that most of their colleagues were far from understanding and accepting the new curriculum. Because more faculty members were needed to serve as tutors and preceptors, a concerted effort would be required to bring them into this new culture.[11] A member of the committee, C. Roland Christensen, described the "teaching practice culture" that had developed at the Harvard Graduate School of Business Administration as faculty came to understand that teaching must be centered on the learner if they wanted to graduate students with a capacity to lead and to act responsibly, to deal with situations effectively, to apply knowledge in practice, and to be lifelong learners.[12] According to Christensen, in order to be successful in this new culture faculty need both an understanding of educational theory and new skills for putting it into practice. The committee recommended that faculty skills-training seminars and workshops begin immediately, facilitated by specialist consultants and offering faculty members first-hand experience in the full span of educational methods proposed for the New Pathway project.

Throughout 1984 and 1985 the faculty development subcommittee continued to study the implications of the new curriculum on faculty in order to identify anticipated needs. Their work culminated in a report to the Harvard Medical School Conference of Department Heads and the Faculty Council containing two major recommendations.

First, a faculty development program should be established to serve the instructional needs of New Pathway faculty members. The program should address the knowledge, skills, and attitudes needed by teachers and include orientation sessions, meetings of the teaching faculty, seminars and workshops, and expert assistance to individual teachers. These activities should be coordinated and carried out under the guidance of a professional educator.

Second, a system for documenting and evaluating the educational scholarship and practice of New Pathway faculty should be established. Evaluation of teaching should be understood by all faculty to be a required part of participation in the new courses and should be linked clearly to opportunities for feedback and improvement. Evidence of teaching accomplishments of New Pathway faculty should be documented in a standard protocol and communicated to department chairs. For this purpose, the Committee on New Pathway Teaching should be formed. This group would be responsible for designing a teaching portfolio system and serving as a source of peer review when an individual was recommended by his or her academic department for promotion. In the appointments and promotions process, the weighting of the various elements of a faculty member's contribution should be sufficiently flexible to accommodate, indeed encourage, greater emphasis on the teaching component than had traditionally been the case in the medical school.

Establishing a Faculty Development Program

Funding from the President of Harvard University, Derek Bok, supported a new program to assist faculty in the development of teaching skills appropriate for the New Pathway project and to focus attention on the importance of teaching excellence for all of Harvard Medical School.

Given the fundamental modifications in the learning opportunities offered to medical students in the New Pathway project—a significant reduction in the number of lectures and widespread use of a small-group tutorial format—initial faculty development efforts were focused on increasing the faculty's awareness and understanding of problem-based theory.[13] Once they were aware of the possibilities, faculty members were persuaded to participate. In the New Pathway program, the most persuasive evidence came from the students themselves, either from testimony or from actual performance in tutorial. Almost as powerful was the opportunity to be a "student" in a tutorial using a case that sparked a personal interest in learning. Colleagues also provided evidence of the impact of problem-based learning by reporting personal experience, testifying to degree of student achievement, or comparing learning outcomes with previous teaching experience in the traditional curriculum. After making a decision to adopt the innovation, faculty members needed individual assistance to develop the necessary knowledge and skills.

For those faculty members who volunteered to become involved early in the process of innovation, the first three steps—knowledge, persuasion, decision—had already been accomplished. Faculty development efforts then focused on building skills. In recruiting beyond the initial volunteers during a period of broad expansion of the innovation, faculty development programs addressing knowledge, persuasion, and decision-making assumed primary importance. Although these goals were partially addressed in group settings, they required a great deal of individualized assistance in order to facilitate an actual decision to adopt.

Principles for Designing a Faculty Development Program

We used several principles in designing faculty development programs for the New Pathway courses and clerkships. This section delineates these principles and describes examples of programs growing out of their application.

Principle 1. Faculty need to understand the educational philosophy of the New Pathway project, with its emphases on an integrated view of basic and clinical sciences, the use of meaningful problems as a focus of the curriculum, students' responsibility for learning, a biopsychosocial model of medicine, and the development of students' ability to reason with and apply knowledge. Programs should include an introduction to these concepts. In a study of effective tutoring conducted at the University of New Mexico's Primary Care Curriculum program, students and faculty concurred that the most effective tutors, lecturers, and preceptors understand the principles of the curriculum.[14]

New preceptors in the Patient–Doctor course attend a daylong faculty development conference at the beginning of the fall semester. The goals of the conference are to introduce student-directed learning methods while reinforcing the psychosocial model of care around which the course is built. Faculty members gather in a small group for the entire day to examine course materials, their own teaching skills, and their approach to history-taking. As a team, they interview a patient at bedside, set up and conduct a feedback session, run a practice tutorial, manage a role-playing exercise, or question a panel of experienced preceptors. Later in the day the teams are joined by facilitators who encourage group members to set their own goals, assess their own performance, and teach one another. At the end of the day participants reflect on their experiences as members of a small student-directed group and gain new insights into the nature of the group experience and the differences between Socratic and student-centered discussion. The workshop methods mirror the philosophy of the curriculum, thereby providing both a verbal description of and an experience in problem-based learning.

Principle 2. Learning is more likely to occur when faculty members perceive a need for new information, skills, or attitudes.[15] Therefore, faculty development programming should grow out of needs identified by the faculty. Planning should include interviews with faculty and course directors as well as direct observation of teaching.[16]

After tutoring for one year, faculty members attend a daylong Conference for Experienced Tutors. The program is based on a survey of all tutors for workshop ideas and volunteers.[17] For example, in 1988 those who returned the survey (42 percent) indicated a need for workshops on teaching problem-solving and reasoning more explicitly, promoting synthesis and conceptual understanding, responding to interpersonal conflict, and diagnosing academic and study problems. The resulting conference offered sessions on the following topics:

- Teaching problem-solving and reasoning more explicitly
- Managing interpersonal conflict
- Diagnosing academic problems
  - Cognitive behavior of strong and weak learners
  - Helping students with study strategies
- The impact of individual differences on the tutorial group
  - Gender differences
  - Cultural differences
  - Dental students
- Promoting synthesis and conceptual understanding
- Encouraging students to take responsibility for the group

Principle 3. Because the problem-based tutorial is applied somewhat differently in each course as the content to be learned shapes the ways in which cases are encountered and discussed, faculty may be better able to appreciate the power of this method of learning if faculty development occurs in the context of their own courses. Through use of actual course materials they can experience how these cases stimulate learning of the concepts and skills that they value. Offering programs in the context of a specific course also provides an opportunity for faculty to share content expertise and to develop a teaching community around shared experiences.

Becoming a problem-based tutor involves individual and group activities before, during, and after the course in which one teaches. All of these activities, which include tutor training, case review, individual feedback discussions, and faculty development workshops, might involve about twenty-five hours for a new tutor in addition to actual teaching time.

Janet Hafler, a faculty development specialist, leads several tutor activities for the first-year course Metabolism and Function of the Human Organ Systems. Four months before the start of the course, in tandem with the course directors, she speaks individually with each of the new tutors, asking them why they decided to tutor, what their perceptions are about the nature of the program, how it meshes with their own views on learning, and what teaching skills they perceive as important for the problem-based tutor. These interviews enable Janet to get acquainted with the faculty as individuals, to assess the accuracy of their understanding of the New Pathway philosophy and begin to address their individual fears and concerns, and to answer questions from them about the program.

Janet encourages the new tutors to visit a tutorial in the current first-year course and to talk with the tutor and students afterward. In addition, she sends them a copy of *The Tutorial Experience,* a handbook written by second-year students in the class of 1990 for their incoming colleagues.[18] The guide describes the tutorial process and details strategies for students to use in facilitating discussion among all members of the group, with special comments on understanding cultural and gender differences.

One month before the course begins, the new tutors attend the first of two faculty development sessions. They hear from experienced tutors and students and serve as "learners" in a simulated tutorial using a case from the course. The simulated tutorials are led by teams of experienced tutors and educators and include time for discussion of the case and of the discussion process. This exercise provides a model for the tutorial format and an opportunity to experience its power as a learning strategy.

In the second workshop, two weeks before the course begins, faculty members are introduced to the role of the tutorial in the course, including a quick overview of each case used and its coordination with concurrent lectures and laboratories. The author of the first case answers questions about the basic science and clinical issues raised. Finally, since they are not expert in all the topics addressed by the cases, new tutors are offered a choice of course textbooks or a clinical textbook to use in their own preparation for the tutorial.

During the course the tutors meet weekly to preview the upcoming cases with expert colleagues. Familiarity with the content and learning objectives of a case has been demonstrated to influence the number of learning issues identified by students, their congruence with case-writer goals, and the time students spend in individual study.[19] For the new tutors, this is also an opportunity to seek informal advice from colleagues on the tutorial process and to develop a sense of confidence, collegiality, and commitment to the course.[20] Most tutors attend these sessions on a regular basis.

Starting in the third week of the course, Janet observes a tutorial led by each of the new tutors and provides individual feedback. These conversations begin with the tutor's own assessment of the experience and then range widely over student accomplishments, teaching strategies, the use of the case, the choice of resources for study, and the appropriate balance of listening and contributing for this group. This is the first time that most tutors have received this kind of individual feedback on their teaching from a colleague.

At the end of the course the Committee on Educational Evaluation asks students to rate the course, the cases, the tutor, and other instructors in the course. Ratings are summarized for each faculty member and returned to the course directors for distribution. Before disbanding for the year, the course faculty meet to discuss changes in cases and to offer suggestions for improvement.

Two indirect sources of data provide some idea of the impact of faculty development activities. First, student ratings of the overall performance of their tutors are high, with 87 percent of those responding in 1987–88 giving their tutors a rating of 1 (excellent) or 2 (good) on a five-point scale.[21] Second, the fact that the majority of tutors return suggests that they achieve some measure of comfort with problem-based learning, the philosophy, the course content, and the tutorial method.

Principle 4. Although large-group workshops are useful for raising consciousness and introducing teaching skills, their most powerful contribution is the opportunity they provide for faculty to work together and learn from one another. This opportunity for colleagueship seems to be a major reason for faculty's willingness to participate in the New Pathway project.[22] Workshops should always provide for active participation and the exchange of ideas among faculty. Typically, faculty development workshops offered as part of the Conference for Experienced Tutors combine opportunities for small-group problem-solving, role-playing, and large-group discussion along with brief presentations of new educational concepts or teaching strategies.[23]

Principle 5. Intensive teaching-skill development comes through actual participation in a problem-based course accompanied by opportunities for feedback from students, review of videotapes of sessions, or direct observation and feedback by a peer or an educational consultant. Although this is a resource-intensive approach to faculty development, research on skill acquisition suggests that practice and feedback are essential ingredients in the change process.[24]

Principle 6. The diversity of their schedules and locations makes getting faculty together difficult. The larger the group, the harder it is to find a convenient time. Smaller gatherings on multiple occasions with multiple sites increase the chance of involving those central to the teaching program, especially clinical faculty.

The New Pathway clinical clerkship in ambulatory care places a student with a single internal medicine preceptor for two clinical sessions a week over a two-month period. As the clerkship moved from the status of a pilot to that of a requirement for the entire class, the development of new preceptors was essential. A centrally held workshop on ambulatory teaching attracted a minority of the new preceptors, mostly those already skilled in the process. Linda Lesky, a clinician educator, Allan Goroll, an experienced preceptor, and I developed a three-phase program of preceptor development that we have taken "on the road." An initial two-hour workshop is held at one of the ambulatory sites to introduce four common teaching dilemmas in precepting students, using a series of multiple-station exercises (Objective Structured Teaching Exercise) based on the concept of the Objective Structured Clinical Examination.[25] During the workshop each preceptor has ten minutes to address and resolve the teaching dilemma raised in each station. For example, in one station the preceptor is asked to give feedback to a student who has not been able to conduct an initial history within the thirty-minute framework previously suggested by the preceptor. At the end of the four stations, the preceptors meet with the students who participated in the various stations and the faculty development staff to discuss precepting difficulties and possible solutions.

In addition to raising awareness of important teaching skills, the stations provide baseline data for assessing the impact of the faculty development program that follows. After the on-site workshop, new preceptors are invited to participate in a teaching laboratory scheduled at their own convenience. In this three-hour follow-up session, the preceptor has the opportunity to supervise and teach a fourth-year student who is seeing patients at the Massachusetts General Hospital in the Primary Care Practice under the guidance of Allan Goroll. Patient–student–preceptor interactions are videotaped for self-review and discussion with Dr. Goroll, who provides structure and feedback throughout the experience. Several months after completing their precepting assignment, the faculty members are invited to a second round of teaching stations, this time with individual feedback from the participating students.

The strategies for precepting promoted in this series of faculty development activities focus on combining teaching with patient care and promoting students' responsibility for meaningful learning. In particular, preceptors are encouraged to set clear expectations for the clinical experience, to identify and build on student needs, to ask students to recommend diagnostic and treatment decisions rather than simply observe, and to give specific feedback that takes into account the student's perspective.[26]

Faculty response to the multiple-station exercise, laboratory experience, and student feedback has been positive. Preceptors have found different aspects of the program most helpful and have appreciated the opportunity for individualized assistance and feedback.

Principle 7. Faculty often speak more powerfully to one another than do the most skilled educational consultants. Social learning theory suggests that role models perceived to be of high status are powerful tools for learning.[27] The participation of such faculty in planning and implementing faculty development activities enhances the credibility and usefulness of the programs. Students can also provide insights into the problem-based learning process in a way that others cannot and should be involved in programming as well.

During the initial offering of new problem-based courses, tutor "press conferences" provided an excellent mechanism for new tutors to learn about the role of the tutor from more experienced colleagues. The exchange among members of the panel and the "press" were lively and the tutors' "pearls" invaluable in understanding both the process of tutorial learning and requisite teaching skills. As we expanded to include the entire class, Dean Tosteson invited tutors from each new course to discuss their reactions to the new curriculum with him over a leisurely lunch. Tutors had a chance to compare perspectives and to hear the commitment of the dean to more active forms of learning.

In the first course of the New Pathway curriculum, the Human Body, tutors play an essential role in introducing the students to the demands of self-directed learning. One of the course directors writes about one of the key skills needed by tutors in this course:

> *Listening.* As you are aware, the most important function we provide in the tutorial setting is extremely careful listening. There are six generalizations about what to listen for. (1) Listen for content, logic, substantive facts, intellectual information. This is what is most obvious. (2) Listen for continuity. Listen over time. Remember who said what, and in what context, so that you can direct back to what was said. Listening over time allows you to observe change. (3) Listen for assumptions *crucial* for arguments but left unstated. (4) Listen for emotion. Listen for *certitude:* are absolutes or conditionals used? Listen for depth of feeling, voice tone, spoken words, latent feelings. (5) Listen to mechanics. Which words are spoken loudly, which ones are mumbled? (6) Listen for a person's capacity to listen.

Rewarding Teaching

Although faculty members have cited the opportunity for in-depth contact with students and collaboration with peers as rewards for New Pathway teaching, Dean Tosteson recognized the need to provide institutional rewards for teaching as well.[28] Since 1983 several committees had been studying the institutional response to teaching contributions. As a result, a new set of criteria for promotion, the Teacher-Clinician criteria, was approved in May 1988.

An examination of the transition from a system in which promotion was occasionally awarded to a stellar teacher (who also did acceptable research) to one in which clinical educational excellence ensures full access to appointment, promotion, a full undifferentiated title, and appointment of unlimited duration elicits several key strategies for change. First, the personal and professional development of faculty was linked with the operation and design of the New Pathway project from the beginning. The committee on faculty development was appointed by Dean Tosteson in 1983, two years before the first students were admitted to the New Pathway pilot. The importance of the committee was evident in the selection of Dean Daniel Federman as chairman and the inclusion of senior, well-respected, and influential faculty. Their final report was distributed and discussed widely among faculty groups and department heads in the spring of 1985.

Second, the committee's report delineated a clearly structured system that could be used by departmental and schoolwide promotion committees for the assessment of teaching. The recommendations, though specific to Harvard University, offer valid general guidelines[29] for any institution developing a teaching evaluation system:

1. The evaluation of teaching should be accepted by all faculty members who plan to teach in the new curriculum.
2. Evaluation policies must be explicitly stated and clearly conveyed to the faculty.
3. The faculty should be assisted in developing their skills as teachers through the establishment of a faculty development program.
4. The evaluation system should include numerous perspectives on teaching excellence (for example, teaching effectiveness, educational scholarship, leadership) and utilize multiple data sources (for example, student assessment of teaching quality, evidence of educationally relevant scholarship, self-report of teaching quantity, and peer review of quality and appropriateness of content).
5. The evidence of teaching accomplishments of New Pathway faculty members should be documented in a standard protocol (a teaching portfolio) that can be used in the promotion process.
6. A faculty development and evaluation resource group should be made responsible for receiving, assessing, and reporting to appropriate department heads the documentation of the educational scholarship and teaching performance of New Pathway faculty.
7. The appointments and promotions process of the medical school should be sufficiently flexible to accommodate, indeed encourage, greater emphasis on the teaching component than has traditionally been the case at this school.

Third, implementation of these recommendations was not left to chance. The New Pathway project core faculty appointed a resource committee to formulate, collect, and assess the teaching portfolios of its faculty as described in the report. In 1987 this committee began to collect documentation on teaching effort and quality from the initial years of the New Pathway project. After two years, portfolios were summarized and reviewed by the committee and reports on teaching quantity and quality written to respective department heads.

Fourth, the changes accomplished in the New Pathway pilot group laid the groundwork for reform of the promotion system of the medical school. In the fall of 1987, when two powerful department chairmen expressed concern that the clinical faculty who supported their departments' clinical and educational efforts were not able to advance beyond the academic level of instructor in the present system, Dean Tosteson had a position paper prepared on evaluating teaching for discussion with department heads and the faculty governing body. After initial approval of the concept, the Teacher-Clinician Task Force, headed by Lee Goldman, recommended that new criteria for appointment and promotion be formulated to recognize full-time faculty serving as teachers of clinical disciplines. These new criteria were to be equal in rigor and title to existing traditional criteria for laboratory and clinical investigators. Guidelines for entry and promotion under the proposed criteria were outlined by the committee and approved for implementation by the faculty in June 1988.

Once again, implementation was not left to chance. The Teacher-Clinician Committee on Education was formed of senior faculty renowned for their educational leadership, an academic dean, and an educator. Over the next year this committee created guidelines for preparing a teaching portfolio that would include self-report of teaching effort, examples of educationally relevant scholarship, student evaluations of teaching effectiveness, and peer assessment of educational contributions. In May 1989 Joan, whose story was presented earlier in this chapter, was promoted to assistant professor after nine years as an instructor.

Looking to the Future

Faculty development and evaluation continue to be interdependent and complementary. Evaluation assesses current levels of teaching performance and identifies strengths and deficits; development assists faculty in improving skills and in learning to use new teaching modalities. It is the responsibility of the institution to provide resources for nurturing the professional competencies on which its faculty are to be judged.

Faculty development and evaluation are not activities to be undertaken only during a period of curricular reform. Faculty must sustain and nurture an innovation. In turn, they must be sustained and nurtured in their own development as educators. To this end Harvard Medical School established an Office for Educational Development, staffed collaboratively by professional educators, basic scientists, and clinicians to provide guidance to the educational program, to assist in continued evaluation of the curriculum, and to stimulate excitement about the process of teaching and learning.

Rewarding teaching also requires sustained institutional commitment. Recognizing that in the New Pathway project personal rewards accrue from teaching, it is incumbent on the medical school to make teaching in the program both possible and desirable with tangible, though small, financial incentives and assistance in making the work easier and more fun. In addition, the Teacher-Clinician Committee on Education continues to be involved in disseminating information on the new promotion criteria, assisting faculty in compiling portfolios, and encouraging attention to the educational mission of the medical school throughout Harvard University.

In summary, faculty development and evaluation programs have contributed significantly to the process of curricular change at Harvard Medical School. A continued institutional commitment to these areas is essential to the maintenance of educational innovations, particularly those like problem-based learning that require a substantial investment of faculty time and creative energy for their implementation.

7

Information Technology

G. Octo Barnett
with Judith L. Piggins, Wayne Raila,
Robert A. Jenders, Henry C. Chueh,
and Bruce Forman

"Life is short, the art long, occasion instant, experiment perilous, decision difficult"—these ancient words from Hippocrates are carved in stone on one of the walls in the Harvard Medical School quadrangle. Given the state of medical education today, we might well want to revise this statement to include the words: "books innumerable, journals countless, lectures endless."

In the last four decades we have witnessed an information explosion in medical knowledge. The quantity and complexity of new scientific knowledge in the basic medical sciences and in the development of new methods for the diagnosis and treatment of illness make keeping abreast of the medical knowledge base a formidable task. This rapid expansion of knowledge has placed impossible time demands on the curriculum. It has been estimated that over 600,000 articles are published in the biomedical literature each year. Even if the most conscientious student attempted to keep up with the literature by reading 2 articles per day, in one year he or she would be over 800 years behind. Many medical educators and most students feel overwhelmed by information overload. Typically students perceive that they are presented with far more information than time in which to master it; most of the time, they feel their education is like trying to get a drink of water from a fire hydrant. Unfortunately, increasing the duration of professional education is not practical, increasing the fragmentation that results from narrow specialization is not wise, and depending on continuing education to fill the gap is simply not possible.

Comprehensive training and experience with modern methods of information management during students' education and training may greatly enhance their effectiveness as health care practitioners and their professional commitment to lifelong learning and teaching. The practice of medicine is intrinsically dependent on how physicians process, record, retrieve, and communicate information. Information technology has the potential to facilitate the mastery of the ever-changing and ever-broadening knowledge concerning the etiology, prevention, and treatment of disease as well as the maintenance of health.

In 1984 Harvard Medical School received the first of several generous grants from the Hewlett Packard Company. These grants have supported an extensive effort to use computer technology in medical education applications. There are now more than 350 personal computers in the Medical Education Center, the Countway Library, the medical school dormitory, the teaching hospitals affiliated with Harvard Medical School, and the homes and offices of students, faculty, and staff.

This chapter outlines our use of information technology in the New Pathway over the past decade. We appreciate that these interpretations and conclusions must be made within the context of our particular experience. We also are aware that such interpretations must be made within the context of time, because of the fast-changing nature of the technology, and because both our faculty and students are rapidly developing a much greater knowledge, experience, and understanding of the potential and the issues in the use of information technology.

Selection of Hardware and Software

For a large institution, selecting technology that offers appropriate capabilities for a wide variety of applications and compatibility with equipment already in place is extraordinarily difficult. The problems are compounded by lack of standardization and rapid evolution in both hardware and software. There are only three options: delay a decision in the hope that the technology will stabilize; replace old technology yearly with the latest, most powerful equipment available; or select one computer system and exploit this technology for several years, ignoring newer, more promising technologies that become available in the meantime. We chose the third approach as the least unsatisfactory compromise and found that a particular hardware platform has a useful software support life of about three to five years. As a result of the generous grant from the Hewlett Packard Company, most of our experience has been based on its Vectra computers (using first the Intel 80286, and more recently the 80386 and 80486 microprocessors), with applications written in a variety of languages using either the MS-DOS or Windows operating system. We have found this a powerful and reliable technical environment that enabled us to provide an integrated set of applications with a relatively standard user interface (including complex graphic displays and computer-controlled videodisks). In the last few years the medical school has acquired a number of Macintosh computers that are used in a similar fashion in medical educational applications.

The choice of computer programs to use in a medical educational application is not simple. There are an increasing number of educational programs that can be obtained from different sources, although it is time-consuming and often frustrating to identify attractive possible candidates for evaluation. The quality of such programs varies greatly, and rarely does the faculty know what programs are currently available in a particular discipline or whether a particular program is of appropriate quality or could be easily integrated with the content of the curriculum. In addition, the two different types of hardware (Vectra MS-DOS and Macintosh) available for curricular use create a problem in that many educational programs are available for only one platform. We have found that personnel costs and technical complexity are significantly increased by the requirement to duplicate a particular educational application on both platforms, to provide a common user interface to the same application, or to provide a seamless integration of applications on the different platforms. Even among software programs that are supported on both hardware configurations, there tend to be marked differences in styles of presentation and methods of interaction. Because of these limitations, we have concentrated on developing most of our own educational applications, focusing on meeting the unique needs of Harvard Medical School students and exploiting the technical and educational opportunities identified by our faculty. Although we have tried whenever possible to provide a common interface and a common method of user interaction with the computer programs to minimize unnecessary student learning effort, a number of applications are available on only one of the hardware platforms.

Integration into the Curriculum

Our strategy for introducing information technology into the curriculum was initially to provide computer applications for use by the students on an ad hoc basis. We chose this approach believing that if the applications were worthwhile, students would seek out and take advantage of the resource. We became increasingly aware, however, of two fundamental weaknesses in this approach.

First, the demands of the medical curriculum are so intense that many students must struggle just to keep up with what faculty identify as essential, ignoring activities with less bearing on their evaluation. Typically, the criterion for judging a software application's usefulness is whether its use is required for passing or doing well in a course.

Second, faculty responsible for course design tend not to invest time and effort in the development, installation, and promotion of computer applications unless and until such applications are explicitly identified as essential components of the curriculum. There is little research that shows conclusively that computers are superior to, or can replace, traditional methods of learning. Without such proof, administrators and faculty are reluctant to abandon traditional methods and tend to view computer-aided tools as an optional resource. In the crowded medical curriculum, this usually means that computer-based resources are used suboptimally. As a result of our experience we now believe that if the full potential of the medical educational application of information technology is to be achieved, computer applications must be a required supplement to regular curricular materials and, where possible, explicitly replace some traditional curricular activities.

Computer-based medical educational applications must offer advantages beyond the use of paper texts. Using a computer program often requires more effort than consulting a textbook or course notes; often a student must take time to go to a place where the appropriate machine is located and learn to use the interface of a particular application. Therefore, the computer-based tool must offer distinct advantages that compensate for the extra effort. In general, students enthusiastically support case simulations that vary the content of the cases, since such clinical problem-solving is perceived as helpful in preparing for clinical rotations and since no textbook can offer such a feature. Students also value programs that make intensive use of graphics and visual images.

Courseware Development

Developing high-quality educational applications demands a great deal of time and effort from faculty and technical staff, even with the aid of authoring tools. Planning how a subject should be presented, generating the appropriate text, and collecting appropriate graphics are very time-consuming. Incorporating other media such as graphics or video offers new opportunities for educational presentation and interaction but adds correspondingly to the intellectual process of creating the programs as well as to their technical complexity.

In addition to the large time commitment required, several other reasons make it difficult to recruit faculty for courseware development. Many faculty members are not familiar with computer technology and are not particularly receptive to the use of computer programs to enhance and supplement learning. In addition, academic institutions do not currently give the same recognition for creating information-technology-based courseware that they do for the publication of articles or books.

Educational Applications

Since 1983 a number of diverse applications have been developed and introduced into the curriculum. Here we discuss only those that represented important opportunities for the development of a technology-based medical educational program beyond the scope of lectures or textbooks.

During the academic year 1988–89 a committee of faculty and staff studied the use of computers in medical education at the medical school and made recommendations about the future use of computers in the curriculum. The committee advised that the core curriculum be designed to include training to assure competency in four major areas.

1. Basic skills: word processing, electronic mail, bibliographic searching, spreadsheets, and database languages

2. Data management: use of collections of data, both individual ones created by each user (for example, a personal reference file of facts or references) and existing databases such as Medline
3. Knowledge management: biological and physiological simulation programs, patient simulations, and browsing programs for textual or graphic information
4. Decision support systems: applications that support clinical decision-making, such as the DXplain program, which uses a medical knowledge base to suggest possible diagnoses for a specified set of signs and symptoms

In the early years of the New Pathway project much effort was devoted to developing computer programs that supported the basic skills. These technical resources are now mature and are supported by the Office for Educational Services and the medical school library as part of their routine operations. Word processing, bibliographic searching, and electronic mail facilities are now widely available. The major developmental focus of the information technology staff has now shifted to data management, knowledge management, and decision support systems.

Word Processing

In the initial years of the New Pathway project, word processing was viewed as an advanced technology with which few students had experience. In addition, there was little support by the faculty for emphasizing this skill as an important educational resource. Over time there have been major changes in both areas. Most students now come to medical school with extensive experience in word processing and virtually demand technical support for this resource as an essential aspect of the educational environment. In 1990 the Curriculum Committee required that all student write-ups of patient contacts be done in electronic format, starting in the first year Patient–Doctor course. This requirement was readily accepted by the students.

Bibliographic Retrieval

Any curriculum that aims to promote the importance of lifelong learning must provide instruction in accessing and using published materials. Each month more than 3,000 journals containing more than

17,000 articles are indexed by the National Library of Medicine. This institution's computer-based database (MEDLINE) is available via dial-up service as well as through commercial vendors (for example, CD-Plus, BRS/Colleague, PaperChase) and on electronic media, such as compact disks for local use on personal computers. The Countway Library supports bibliographic access with a local, frequently updated copy of CD-PLUS. Since 1989 Harvard Medical School students have been instructed in computer-based searching and are required to carry out literature searches as part of laboratory exercises in various courses.

Electronic Mail

Electronic mail allows an individual to use a network of computers to exchange messages with other users over either a communications network or standard telephone lines. Messages can be directed to a specific individual or simultaneously to several users or can be posted to an electronic bulletin board for any reader. Because of the geographic dispersion of the Harvard Medical School faculty, this application has proved to be immensely helpful in curriculum planning and development and in communicating with other faculty and students about specific course questions. Students use the system for sharing ideas about the curriculum assignments, personal interactions, and questioning the faculty. When the New Pathway was extended to the entire student body, access to electronic mail was primarily through computers located in the Medical Education Center, and the use of electronic mail decreased sharply. Only in recent years has student usage begun to increase to the previous levels. Many students also use the Internet capabilities supported by the Harvard Medical School network to communicate with faculty supervisors and with colleagues at Harvard and at other schools across the nation.

Computer-Based Simulations

In our experience the most popular and effective computer-based educational programs are those that are highly interactive, use visual and graphic material, and involve the student in active problem-solving. Using both the Vectra MS-DOS and Macintosh technology, we have developed a number of computer-based simulations to help students acquire medical knowledge, understand how complex body systems function and interact, and learn clinical judgment and patient care decision-making skills. We are using computer simulations of biological systems to emulate the laboratory environment so that students may observe realistic models in a variety of states, introduce different interventions, and learn by trying "what-if" experiments. Computer-simulated models also allow instructors to control the experiment more explicitly.

One of the physiological simulations developed for the New Pathway project involves acid–base regulation in which students learn to characterize a variety of acid–base abnormalities. This program makes use of the color graphics capability of the Vectra to illustrate the effects of clinical interventions on the acid–base balance of a simulated patient, as well as providing general background and explanatory material at the student's request. The acid–base program has been used both in courses and in independent study.

The New Pathway also uses computer-based clinical simulations to help students learn the techniques of clinical problem-solving, which often involve complex and sequential decision-making. Students must acquire the critical cognitive skills involved in deciding what information to collect. They must also determine when there are sufficient data to justify making a diagnosis and then select the appropriate therapy. Despite the importance of clinical judgment in medical practice, clinical training consists primarily of a series of graded apprenticeships in which there is little systematic attempt to provide explicit models of the intellectual processes involved in medical decision-making. For the most part, students are expected to acquire clinical judgment by learning to imitate the patterns of their instructors.

This time-honored way of teaching has several potential weaknesses. First, each student's educational experience is relatively unstructured and may be incomplete. Second, skilled teachers with adequate time for close student supervision may not be available. Third, there may not be an optimal mix of patient cases available for each student to learn about various disease entities.

In a computer-based patient simulation, the student acts the role of the doctor, and the computer acts the role of the patient. The student controls the dialogue, asking questions to ascertain signs and symptoms and laboratory test results, developing and testing hypotheses, and making management decisions. The "patient" responds to the questions and therapeutic decisions in a manner congruent with the underlying disease process.

There are obvious limitations to the computer-based simulations. Because it is necessary to reduce the variability of real life to fit the computer model, the "patient case" is far more simplistic than would be true in real life. Also, the computer program is unable to elicit or measure the patience and compassion that a doctor must exhibit in responding to a patient's questions and anxieties. Despite these limitations, there are major advantages in supplementing clinical training with computer-based simulations. Many students learn best through trial and error, using the "what-if" approach. They can practice and make mistakes without danger or inconvenience to real patients. They can learn the effects of particular interventions by "experience" rather than by simply reading or being told about the particular tactic. In addition, they can see and "manage" a greater number of patient cases and a variety of diseases. The program provides guidance on request in the form of a "consultant" who advises on additional items of information that would be useful to gather. Once the correct diagnosis has been made, the program allows the student to specify how the patient should be managed. On completion of a case, a critique of the student's performance is given, indicating how efficient the workup was in terms of the relevance and cost of the items of information requested.

We have developed and support a large variety of computer-based simulations on topics ranging from the differential diagnosis of abdominal pain to cardiopulmonary arrest and the classification of a cardiac arrhythmia. Several pathophysiology patient-case simulations have been developed in the Macintosh environment by Dr. Robert A. Greenes and the Decision Systems Group at the Brigham and Women's Hospital. Most of these simulations are used on an ad hoc basis and have proved especially popular with second-year students as they begin to have patient contact and make the transition from textbook disease descriptions to the uncertainties and ambiguities of diagnostic problem-solving when the diagnosis is not known. The Vectra-based simulations are also used in the clinical years (years III and IV), providing students with experience in specific disease categories as well as honing general clinical decision-making skills. A modified version of these programs was used in evaluating student learning under the new curriculum format versus the traditional format.

Knowledge Access Incorporating Visual/Graphic Presentation

Disciplines such as medicine require acquisition of an entirely new knowledge base: a new vocabulary, a great many new facts, and a collection of new rules. The amount of rote learning required is one of the elements of medical education that many students find most distasteful. Lectures and reading are useful approaches to learning detailed factual information but may not be sufficiently stimulating to result in effective long-term recall.

We have developed several applications in both the Vectra and Macintosh environments to present information in a visually oriented, problem-solving context. With commercially available technology for microcomputers, one can now easily display high-resolution videodisk and digital images with computer-generated text and graphics. Thus, one can present an image and simultaneously overlay explanatory text or graphic highlights for clarification. The program can highlight items in the image, and the user can interact with the program by using a mouse to point at features of the image.

One example is a required supplement in the anatomy block. This module integrates organ-specific material from gross anatomy and CAT scan images in a structured, problem-solving, interactive program that acquaints students with cross-sectional, radiographic anatomy. The objective is to introduce and reinforce concepts of three-dimensional relationships among organs and the topography of the normal abdomen. CAT scans are integrated and coordinated with anatomical drawings. Navigation is facilitated by mouse interactions with "hot" text or "hot" graphics/video regions and integrated pull-down menus.

Another visually oriented module allows students to focus on a single organ system (the kidney) and "browse" through pertinent facts from anatomy, biochemistry, physiology, and pharmacology for each high-resolution image. The objective is to enhance integration of basic sciences content in the context of the organ system being studied.

In these computer-based exercises the computer can act as a responsive tutor, carrying on an interactive dialogue with the student, who is challenged to think and respond rather than to read or listen passively to a set of facts. Students maintain control over the interaction and use the program at their own pace, exploring the capabilities of the system in whatever sequence is of interest. This use of the computer cannot substitute for the presence of an inspiring teacher; but it may supplement the teacher's presentation, review, and testing of basic facts and concepts.

Clinical Assessment

One of the major projects now under way in collaboration with senior faculty in charge of the clinical rotations in pediatrics is designed to assess clinical problem-solving skills. The specific objectives of this program are to

- Provide clinical problem-solving challenges that are considered appropriate and relevant by both faculty and students
- Measure predefined problem-solving skills (for example, efficiency of information collection, ability to make appropriate diagnostic interpretations) and clinical knowledge about several different clinical entities
- Provide students with a uniform set of problem-solving patient simulations for each clinical rotation
- Implement scoring and performance evaluation in a defined, predictable, and uniform fashion
- Track student performance closely and produce detailed reports of both individual and aggregate performance

The aim of the program is to provide a more standardized method of student assessment than the heterogeneous and anecdotal protocol currently used in the clinical rotations. The format is similar to that of the patient-based clinical simulations, except that there is more emphasis on formulating presumptive diagnostic hypotheses and on justifying the particular pattern of information items requested during the case. This program should be especially useful in identifying two groups of students: those who demonstrate significant weaknesses in problem-solving and who might benefit from additional remedial assignments, and individuals who demonstrate outstanding clinical problem-solving skills and should be considered for honor grades.

Student Workstations

Keeping medical records is a dominant activity throughout a physician's career, and most experts agree that computers will play an increasingly important role in the recording, retrieval, and analysis of clinical data.

To promote students' appreciation of both the potential and the problems of computer-based medical record systems, we developed a limited computer-based record (Clinical Case Book, CCB) for use in both the initial clinical experience and the clinical rotations. The CCB allows students to use a controlled vocabulary to record the diagnoses and procedures on each patient for whom they have responsibility. These data are collected for each rotation and allow students and faculty to review students' clinical experiences and analyze the actual aggregate of cases seen. Our experience with the CCB has been mixed: a few faculty members are enthusiastic supporters and require its use on their particular rotation; on other rotations, however, there is less faculty support, with the result that few of their students record data in the CCB.

We are currently developing a student workstation that will support a graphic interface and multiple windows for access to information and the creation of an extensive computer-based patient record. This workstation will serve three purposes:

1. Recording of a comprehensive history and physical examination and daily progress notes for each patient for whom the student has clinical responsibility. A combination of controlled structured text and narrative text will be entered by standard keyboard or by a mouse; we are also exploring data entry via voice recognition and pen technology.
2. Access to hospital information systems (particularly databases on laboratory test results) through networking interfaces, data representation, and communication protocols (using standard industry models such as HL-7).
3. Access to reference material through computer-based indexing and retrieval of a variety of computer-based text materials, including a drug database and a bibliographic reference file containing abstracts of current literature. For example, a student recording a physical examination might want more information about a specific aspect of the examination or how to interpret a particular finding such as an abnormal heart sound. Using the workstation, he or she will be able to access this information directly from a computer-stored reference text without resorting to an index or table of contents.

Decision Support

One of the more promising potential applications of information technology is the use of computers to support and facilitate the physician's clinical decision-making activities. In this role, the computer does not replace the physician or the physician's judgment. It can, however, provide immediate access to a large amount of relevant medical information and to a large number of predefined rules of appropriate actions to be taken. Since 1987 a diagnostic clinical decision support program, DXplain, developed and supported by the Laboratory of Computer Science at Massachusetts General Hospital, has been made available to students both on individual personal computers and over the Harvard Medical School communications network. DXplain allows a user to enter a patient's signs and symptoms and then suggests a list of diagnoses consistent with these findings. The list of diagnoses can be refined through additional interaction with the program. The program also provides references and descriptive material on the various diagnoses. A version of the program has been distributed as part of the Countway Library network for use by the Harvard Medical School community.

Cost

The acquisition cost of computer systems continues to decline relative to their power and capability. However, acquisition of new graphics and video technologies (videodisks, CD-ROM, high-resolution graphics systems) tends to add costs, especially when multiple systems must be provided for many students. Also, it must be anticipated that within a few years the equipment will no longer be able to support the newest software and educational applications. These facts discourage administrators in many schools from investing heavily in computer hardware, with the result that only a few computer systems are provided for student use. Lack of ready access to computer technology can significantly limit the value and impact of technological innovations. In our experience, the more constrained access is to computer resources, the less effectively they will be used by students and faculty.

The cost of development (or acquisition) and modification of software is severalfold higher than the initial cost of hardware. This relative difference in cost is increasing each year. Purchasing software from medical publishers or sharing among different medical schools has served only a limited set of needs. Thus far, we have found that our faculty and student requirements demand a major effort in local educational program development.

When software is heterogeneous and changes relatively often, and when computers are used by a large number of relatively naive users at sites located over a wide geographic area, the cost of supporting and maintaining the computer systems over a period of several years can be as large as the initial purchase price. We have found it more difficult to justify expenditure for support, training, and maintenance than for initial acquisition.

Evaluation

Evaluating any innovation in graduate education is difficult, since the students involved have heterogeneous backgrounds and skills, and their academic performance is strongly influenced by factors besides specific changes in curriculum. Evaluation is further complicated by lack of precisely defined goals, primitive and often ambiguous evaluation methodology, and the difficulty of defining and isolating the relevant variables. Evaluation of the information technology innovation in the New Pathway project is particularly difficult because the new curriculum is not concerned specifically with student performance on tests of factual recall. Instead, the goal is to stimulate the students to acquire the total set of skills, attitudes, and knowledge that will result in their becoming competent and caring physicians in careers spanning several decades. Clearly, in this setting a comprehensive and critical evaluation of the impact of information technology would be complex and the results in all likelihood inconclusive.

Thus far, our only specific evaluation of the information technology aspects of the curriculum has been the collection of usage data for the different application programs and of student questionnaires on the usefulness of the different educational modules. These data indicate that most students use the computer systems regularly and that those who do so believe they have a high educational value and would welcome more applications and better integration into the curriculum.

8

Project Evaluation

Susan D. Block and Gordon T. Moore

One reason for the persistence of traditional styles of medical education is the dearth of reliable evaluations of innovative curriculums. For example, many schools have conducted useful studies about problem-based learning, but selection bias and the absence of control groups have limited the conclusions that can be drawn.[1] As a result, medical educators have been unable to provide a comprehensive answer to the question: "What works?"

Design of Project Evaluation

In designing the New Pathway project, we had an opportunity to conduct a program evaluation with a true control group. In the academic years 1985–86 and 1986–87 a larger number of students than could be accommodated applied to be in the new curriculum. From these applicants we randomly selected students for the New Pathway program, assigning equivalent proportions of women and underrepresented minorities to both the new curriculum and a control group, which took the unchanged, traditional curriculum along with a third cohort (called the traditional group) consisting of students who had not applied to be in the new curriculum. This strategy allowed us to reduce self-selection bias as a confounding variable in our evaluation of the impact of the two curriculums. We followed these three groups (New Pathway, control, and traditional) through their years at Harvard Medical School to determine the differences in their educational experiences and to assess how the two curriculums affected their final knowledge, skills, attitudes, and personal characteristics. Most of the students in the two classes proceeded through and graduated from medical school during this project. Sixty-two students were in the New Pathway project, 63 in the control group, and 172 in the traditional group.

Measures

We measured both formative and summative outcomes at points throughout all four years, using a variety of existing and newly developed instruments. We collected demographic information at the beginning and the end of medical school. Surveys carried out at the beginning provided baseline data with which the initial comparability of the three groups could be determined.

Our evaluation focused on student performance and the perceived experience of medical school. Evaluation of performance included biomedical and psychosocial knowledge, clinical reasoning, psychosocial skills and attitudes, and learning styles and preferences. A broad array of instruments was used, including the National Board of Medical Examiners examination Parts I and II; several different measures of clinical reasoning, decision-making processes, diagnostic reasoning, and pattern recognition; clerkship evaluations; self-report instruments regarding personal attitudes and values, orientation to social issues in medicine, intellectual development, locus of control, risk-taking, personality, and moral development; multiple independent measures of student interaction with standardized patients; and measures of cognitive behavior and perceptions of the learning environment. Many of these measures were administered several times to permit comparison of performance over time.

Students' perceived experiences in medical school were studied in an extensive ethnographic project carried out by Byron J. Good and Mary-Jo D. Good, of the Department of Social Medicine and Health Policy at Harvard Medical School. In addition, we administered semistructured interviews at the end of the second and fourth years and a questionnaire during year IV to gain a retrospective view of students' experiences. In the summer of 1993, three to four years after graduation, we used a semistructured interview to ask former New Pathway and control students about their current career plans and their retrospective views of their medical school experience. Overall, we used thirty-four different instruments or measurement approaches over a period of up to eight years.

Student Participation

Student participation in this assessment was entirely voluntary. Despite our emphasis on the importance of the study and offers of individual awards such as books and even a challenge grant for a donation to graduation festivities or a charity of the students' choice, student participation was disappointing. In the first two years participation ranged from almost 100 percent on some measures to a low of 67 percent of eligible New Pathway students and 38 percent of eligible controls on others. Because of both delayed graduation and low participation, some of our observations in the clinical years included as few as 62 percent of New Pathway and 21 percent of control students; on other measures (for example, the National Board of Medical Examiners examination, residency choices, clerkship evaluations), however, response rates were as high as 100 percent of eligible students. Response rates for the follow-up study were approximately 67 percent.

Results

Data collected at orientation demonstrated that students who wanted the New Pathway educational experience (New Pathway students and controls) differed from those who preferred the traditional curriculum in that they entered with higher chemistry and physics Medical College Admission Test (MCAT) subtest scores and showed a higher preference for discovery-style learning. We found no other differences between the New Pathway and the traditional groups on the other measures administered at orientation.

We were unable to demonstrate any significant differences between New Pathway and control students on basic science and biomedical clinical knowledge on the National Board of Medical Examiners examination Parts I and II. New Pathway students, however, scored significantly higher than controls on the behavioral science (Part I) and public health (Part II) subtests. We found no differences between the groups on any measures of clinical reasoning. Medicine clerkship evaluations showed similar levels of clinical performance in students from both groups. In the domain of psychosocial skills and attitudes, by the end of the second year students in the New Pathway project demonstrated stronger interpersonal skills on every measure utilized to evaluate them, and characterized themselves as more comfortable with emotions, more patient-centered, and more tolerant of ambiguity than the controls. In addition, we found significant differences in values associated with "ideal" physicians: more New Pathway students than controls said they valued patient-centeredness and attention to psychosocial issues, and their performance with standardized patients reflected these values. However, we found no differences between the groups in the number of students who took time off while in medical school to pursue research interests.

The limited data we have on performance in the fourth year suggest that while attitudinal differences between New Pathway students and controls were maintained, control students tended to catch up somewhat with New Pathway students in terms of relational skills, and New Pathway students tended to show a marked decline in their previously high level of attention to preventive medicine issues while interviewing patients. The scores of both New Pathway and control students declined dramatically from the second through fourth years on a self-report measure of the importance attached to social factors in medical care. An indirect measure of student values, career choice, suggested significant differences between the two groups: students graduating from the New Pathway program were more likely than controls to elect residencies with high primary care and psychosocial orientation (internal medicine, family practice, pediatrics, and psychiatry).

As expected, learning styles differed between the two groups. Students in the problem-based curriculum preferred a more student-directed learning environment, valued innovation, desired more faculty support, used more reflection, memorized and crammed less, and were lower in their need for clarity than controls. However, by the end of the fourth year both New Pathway and control students were less positive about an unstructured learning environment.

Students in the New Pathway project experienced a greater sense of responsibility for their own education and were more anxious and frustrated than controls in the first two years. Intratutorial group conflicts and the lack of structure regarding what and how much to study were particular sources of strain for the New Pathway group. In the fourth year New Pathway students were significantly more likely to describe their educational experience as "stressful, engaging, and difficult" than control students, who tended to describe their educational program as "nonrelevant, passive, and boring." Finally, in comparison with controls, students in the New Pathway program knew their faculty and were considerably better known to them.

In the follow-up study, former New Pathway students were three times more likely to be in primary care fields than controls, although there was no difference in the number of students planning careers in academic medicine. Reflecting back on their experiences in medical school, New Pathway students generally characterized themselves as better prepared for the psychosocial and ethical challenges of medicine and for ongoing, self-directed learning than controls and, conversely, as having weaker preparation in the basic sciences. Although the strong psychosocial emphasis of the New Pathway project was cited as a major strength of the program, a number of students felt that it was overemphasized. Former New Pathway students also emphasized the importance of relationships with mentors, many of which were still in effect at the end of their residencies. Typical comments were: "I carry with me a wealth of guiding principles that I really live by—I hear them [faculty mentors] giving me advice" and "I remember their [faculty mentors] approaches to problem-solving and model my own thinking on theirs."

These data suggest that participation in the New Pathway educational program was associated with a number of important differences between the New Pathway and control groups that persisted as long as four years after medical school. These differences conform to what might be predicted on the basis of contrasting educational approaches. Compared with students in the traditional curriculum, students in the new curriculum felt more challenged and, at the same time, more uncertain about what and how to study. They used the library and primary and secondary literature more than students in the traditional curriculum. The typical New Pathway student felt better known by the faculty, and many developed long-term relationships with a faculty member with whom they had studied. Students in the new curriculum demonstrated both a more positive orientation to and better knowledge of social and behavioral science, stronger interpersonal skills, and more humanistic attitudes than students in the control group. We found no evidence that the New Pathway experience interfered with acquisition of basic science knowledge.

Limitations of the Study

Some of the more important theoretical advantages of problem-based learning remain unproved. Although we noted some differences in attitudes and performance during medical school, student participation, especially in the fourth-year evaluation, was too low to permit confident generalization about some of these differences. However, the follow-up data, based upon a more representative sample, suggest that some of the attitudinal differences between groups seen during medical school have persisted through residency training. Certainly, the claim that problem-based learning enhances lifelong learning and yields better recall of basic sciences in clinical contexts remains unproved. Longer-term follow-up of students into clinical practice will be necessary to ascertain the impact of the New Pathway curriculum on lifelong learning.

This study taught us firsthand about the difficulty of carrying out performance-based program evaluation. Despite our aspiration to conduct a rigorous, randomized, controlled trial of the New Pathway intervention, our study fell far short of that goal. Many of the difficulties we encountered limit the validity of the conclusions that can be drawn from our data. The problems included limitations of measurement instruments, intergroup interactions that confounded the intervention, measurement bias, and poor participation.

Measurement Instruments

The study was hampered by lack of adequate instruments to measure performance reliably. We often felt that we might be missing important curricular effects because we lacked the tools to measure them. Insofar as the New Pathway project represented a new paradigm for medical education, particularly in the area of the patient–doctor relationship, conventional measurements failed to address the kinds of differences we hypothesized might be generated by the new curriculum. For example, the clinical reasoning measure that we used reflected a conventional biomedical definition of appropriate questions to be asked about clinical data and minimized the potential impact of psychosocial phenomena on the medical problem at hand.

Intergroup Interaction

The New Pathway curriculum and the traditional curriculum were not truly independent interventions. The students in the two groups lived and worked together. Each group obviously knew what was happening in the other program, and tension and competition between the two groups occurred frequently. Each group of faculty tried hard to make its curriculum the best. We believe that the tension between the two curriculums contributed significantly to the low participation rate of students in the traditional curriculum; it certainly had a negative impact on the students' subjective experiences in both curriculums.

Measurement Bias

Students obviously knew which curriculum they were in, so we could not eliminate their conscious bias on performance testing or surveys about the experience. We were more successful in eliminating tester and scorer bias, since we could single-blind evaluators against knowledge of which curriculum each student had taken. We did this whenever possible.

Poor Participation

The most serious limitation was the reluctance of students to be involved in the evaluation project. Participation in the study ranged from 100 percent on some measures to as low as 21 percent on others. Not only do the small numbers limit the significance of demonstrated differences, but nonparticipation undoubtedly introduced bias. In general participation in all assessment procedures was higher among students with better scores on the National Board of Medical Examiners examination. However, there was some suggestion (from the Board's behavioral science subtest) that high-performing New Pathway students and low-performing controls were more likely to participate in the study. This bias would tend to amplify intergroup differences in psychosocial competencies. Furthermore, if it was the angrier students who did not participate, the study, control, and traditional groups may overrepresent those whose experience was more positive and who performed better. It remains possible that biased participation contributed to some of the differences we found, especially in the psychosocial domain.

Our experience enabled us to draw several conclusions about the process of program evaluation. First, unless participation is made mandatory, no study of students is likely to generate adequate numbers and representation. Second, we learned the value of looking for consistent trends across different types of measurement and over time; even small differences, not significant by themselves, took on meaning when they could be fit into an explanatory pattern and when they persisted over time. Finally, we were impressed by the astuteness of participating faculty and students in assessing what they liked and disliked about the new approach.

Our experience suggests that it will be difficult ever to determine conclusively which curriculum is best. Because of selection bias, randomization of students into intervention and control groups is necessary. Only rarely is it possible to conduct a randomized trial of an educational intervention. Poor participation and participation bias, as we encountered here, are common and grow out of the tension that arises when two curriculums are being compared and out of students' reluctance to be evaluated. Reluctant or coerced students are unlikely to offer an accurate indication of their abilities. The measurement of concepts such as "lifelong learning" and "humanism" is extraordinarily complex; although we may get better at defining and measuring these notions over time, it is likely that our measurement abilities will also continue to have weaknesses. Because of these problems, as well as the funding required to conduct research of this complexity and duration, we have concluded that a definitive statement that one curriculum is better than another will be difficult to achieve in the real-life, uncontrolled setting of medical education. In fact, given the difficulty of conducting a conclusive quantitative assessment of any educational method, the students' and faculty's subjective evaluation of the efficacy of curriculum changes may be one of the most powerful, and perhaps the most reliable, methods of assessment.

Conclusions

Our evaluation of the New Pathway curriculum has provided us with no clear indication that it is "better" than the traditional style of medical education, or vice versa. The evaluation did, however, show some important differences and, equally valuable, assured us that this style of learning did not do harm. Students passed examinations, demonstrated strong psychosocial skills, performed well on the wards, showed interest in academic pursuits, matched into good residencies, and continue, three to four years after graduation, to express strong interest in pursuing careers in primary care. Second, the evaluation documented differences in the experience of medical school and demonstrated short-term changes in behavior that reinforce a long-standing practical and theoretical literature stressing the value of student-directed, problem-oriented learning. Third, students generally appreciated the qualities of the New Pathway curriculum even though they did not like all aspects of the experience. We conclude that the New Pathway curriculum yields a few measurable improvements in psychosocial performance, no documentable decrement in traditional knowledge or skill, and some significant enhancements in the quality of students' educational experience.

The ultimate success of any program resides in its capacity to initiate and sustain change. The impressions of faculty who taught in the new curriculum were strongly, though not universally, positive. Since its inception, the curriculum has moved increasingly toward more problem-based, small-group teaching. Where ground was lost in the abandonment of innovations during the transition from the experimental track to a single curriculum, those working on the curriculum have sought ways to restore these innovations. The number of applicants to the school has risen along with the proportion accepting an offered place. Visitors from other medical schools have come in a constant stream to hear about the new curriculum and see it in operation. These indirect measures, though soft, point toward the program's success.

9

The Student Experience

Marc T. Silver

In order to understand Harvard Medical School's experiment, the New Pathway in General Medical Education, one must go beyond the theories and observations of faculty and administrators to the experiences of students, for it is they, more than any other group, who experience the learning facilitated by any teacher in any curriculum. This chapter provides a retrospective overview of students' experience of the New Pathway project in its first four years: how we learned, what we learned, what we did not learn, and how we felt.

What we learned in the New Pathway project was in many ways similar to what students learn in more traditional medical curriculums, at least in terms of the traditional basic and clinical sciences. Indeed, it was not so much the content but the process of the New Pathway that was different. This difference in process, however, changed not only the way we learned but also what we learned. So while we were studying anatomy, physiology, or pharmacology, we were also learning other important things. And at no time during medical school was the way we learned so radically different as in the first two years.

Case-Based Learning

By organizing the entire curriculum of the first two years around real patient cases, the New Pathway project fostered an understanding of the interrelation between the basic and clinical sciences. Basic science was something that had to be comprehended in order to begin to understand a patient and his or her symptoms. Only after gaining acquaintance with the Krebs cycle, insulin, and electrolytes could we understand what diabetic ketoacidosis is and how to help the unconscious patient presented in the case. Only after learning about cell structure and function could we understand how Georgie Markov could die from a tiny dose of diphtheria toxin placed on the tip of an assassin's umbrella. And only after understanding the immune response could we comprehend why patients with AIDS develop opportunistic infections. By so closely integrating the basic and clinical sciences, the designers of the New Pathway project forced us to look at basic science in a totally new way.

Presented with a new "unknown" case at least once a week, we went home to involve ourselves in a process of discovery as we attempted to solve the case. Going home to study was not simply memorizing a pathway, learning a list, or reading an assigned chapter; rather, all of our reading and studying was directed toward answering questions raised by the case or by our tutorial group discussions.

We never viewed the overwhelming number of facts to be learned in basic science as an unnecessary inconvenience, an obstacle placed between medical students and clinical medicine. That is not to say that the amount to be learned in the first two years did not feel overwhelming—it often did. But it never felt superfluous, as it often does to medical students in more traditional curriculums. The necessity of understanding the regulation of blood pressure, the renin-angiotensin-aldosterone system, and the muscles innervated by the radial nerve was never questioned.

The use of patient cases as the center of the New Pathway curriculum was not without problems. While case-based learning made it evident that the basic sciences were indeed the sciences basic to clinical medicine, it also led to a great deal of anxiety. The students who entered the New Pathway project were like any other college graduates entering medical school. We were accustomed to learning from lectures, an occasional teacher-led seminar, and extensive individual studying. Even the last was very directed, however, as the student used required or recommended texts with little leave to determine his or her own learning. In this regard perhaps more than in any other, the New Pathway project differed from more traditional medical school curriculums, leading to a high level of student concern but also to a strong sense of responsibility for one's own learning.

This anxiety was often so intense that it must be listed as a disadvantage of the New Pathway curriculum. Early in the first year it manifested itself in the feeling that we were not learning enough facts, that we were spending too much time talking about clinical medicine, patient–doctor relationships, and group process. We looked at our classmates in the traditional curriculum spending eight hours a day listening to renowned lecturers and reading lecture notes and required textbooks, compared with our one hour of lecture a day, and we felt scared. We seemed to spend a great deal of time trying to figure out what was worth learning as we struggled to set learning agendas in the tutorial groups. We often walked out of these sessions feeling overwhelmed, that our goal in the next forty-eight hours was to learn all of cardiac physiology, all of renal pathophysiology, or the entire anatomy of the upper limb. No wonder we felt anxious.

This anxiety was heightened by the fact that there were definitely "holes," as we came to call them, in the New Pathway curriculum. While it is true that we determined the course of our own learning, the cases played a major role in guiding us. Therefore, if none of the cases stressed biochemical or pharmacologic principles, we would be unlikely to spend much time reading about metabolic pathways or beta blockers. As it turned out, over the first two years as a whole, biochemistry and pharmacology were never introduced in great detail. Although our case on diabetic ketoacidosis forced us to learn some of the metabolic pathways and principles of their hormonal regulation, we were never guided to read about amino acid synthesis. And while patients in many of our cases received a wide variety of drugs, we never had a systematic introduction to the subject of pharmacology.

Many basic scientists and some physicians would look at our curriculum and be dismayed at this state of affairs. Simply looking at the written curriculum design, however, does not give one an understanding of what we actually learned; biochemistry and pharmacology are two examples of this very point. All of us recognized that we were going to end up somewhat deficient in these two traditional subject areas. Partly because we felt them to be important and partly out of fear of not knowing them for the National Board of Medical Examiners examination, we found ways of learning some additional biochemistry and pharmacology. An entirely student-initiated and student-organized case-based elective course in pharmacology was set up with the help of faculty in the Department of Clinical Pharmacology at the Brigham and Women's Hospital. Half of the students in the New Pathway project participated, while others found time to read on their own, and yet others set up independent study electives with various faculty. In the case of biochemistry, an elective course was organized by some New Pathway students, and others arranged independent study electives. In the end, we learned a great deal of biochemistry and pharmacology even though it had not been "given" to us. In those areas where we felt we needed more knowledge, we found ways of obtaining it either as individuals or as a group.

Nonetheless, as Part I of the National Board examination approached, the anxiety level reached a peak. Had the experimental curriculum prepared us for this basic science trivia test? Partly because we were the first group through this new curriculum and partly because no one had ever told us exactly what we needed to know, the weeks before the National Board examination were some of the most stress-filled of the entire four-year experience.

The anxiety, however, always seemed to fade. And with the overcoming of each obstacle our faith grew in our own abilities to set our own learning agendas, to figure out what was important and what was not, and to know when and whom to ask for help. By forcing us to be responsible for our own learning, the New Pathway project taught us to be our own teachers. No one ever told us what we had to learn, where to get the answers, what was important or unimportant. That is not to say that the tutors and lecturers did not help and that the cases did not guide us; rather, our curriculum gave us the message that, in the end, we were responsible for our own learning. As we headed onto the clinical wards in our last two years, we knew how to learn on our own; we were familiar with the journals, the textbooks, the library, the computer search services, and we were not afraid to call upon a professor for help. One of the primary goals of the New Pathway designers had in fact been achieved—we had learned how to learn.

Learning in Groups

The patient cases, the center of the curriculum, were read and discussed in small groups composed of six students and a faculty tutor. These groups themselves became important instruments of learning. Whereas traditional medical curriculums tend to minimize the interaction of students while they are learning, the New Pathway project sought to maximize this interaction. Just as the cases had advantages and disadvantages, so did the tutorial groups.

The disadvantages of learning in groups became apparent quickly. Students did not always get along with one another or with their tutor. Some students and some faculty tutors seemed to dominate the tutorial groups. Some groups were productive and others were less so. The extent to which these disadvantages hindered learning varied from group to group. Although the group experience was realistic in forcing us into situations that were not always ideal, educationally the group occasionally seemed more of a burden than a blessing, especially in the first two years.

Throughout these same years, however, we were often reminded of the advantages of spending a significant amount of time learning in groups. Not infrequently we would enter a tutorial group overflowing with confidence in what we had learned since our last meeting, ready to share our newly acquired knowledge, only to find ourselves unable to answer the probing questions of our peers. Tutorial often served as a painful reminder that you do not understand something until you can teach it to someone else. All too often, what we thought we knew, we knew in only a superficial way. Teaching one another and learning from one another, we were forced to grapple with the material in a highly critical manner. We learned that a quick reading on adrenal function in a physiology textbook does not an endocrinologist make. Only after we had worked through adrenal function in a group, asking tough questions, helping others who did not comprehend, organizing the material on a blackboard, had we taken the first step toward real knowledge.

Learning in groups gave us even more, however: we learned that medicine is filled with uncertainty—indeed, that uncertainty rather than certainty tends to be the norm. Perhaps no achievement of the New Pathway curriculum was more impressive. This acknowledgment of uncertainty had its roots in the group process. After the establishment of the group's learning agenda, each student would consult her or his textbook of choice, supplementing such basic reading with a variety of primary journal sources and going to various experts in the field at the medical school. The group would reconvene at the next tutorial session to discuss what each member had learned. The resulting discussions were often surprising and at times frustrating.

What one student had read in one source had been questioned, or even contradicted, by another source or expert. Given the data available on a given subject, we were often unable to resolve differences of opinion, experimental results, and clinical experiences. We were sometimes left with a mass of uncertainty; more often, however, we were able to understand what was certain and what was not. Sometimes we were forced to consult other books, other texts and journals, other experts. Often we ended up with a fair degree of certainty, but sometimes we did not. The process inevitably left us with more knowledge, better learning skills, and always a realistic understanding of the limits of scientific and medical knowledge.

This process of wrestling with uncertainty led us to interact with faculty at all levels. From these interactions, not to mention the very close and intense interaction with our tutors and others involved in the new curriculum, developed many close student–faculty relationships. These offered students the chance to get to know people in the medical profession in a way different from that offered by the traditional lecture situation. Students were able to find role models, friends, and valuable sources of advice and information. Furthermore, the faculty involved in the New Pathway project were so excited about teaching and learning that they added to the general excitement about learning in groups.

Learning with Computers

The close relationships among students and between students and faculty were enhanced by the computer technology that was a part of the New Pathway project. An electronic mail system linked all students at home and at work with faculty and administrators. Although originally it was hoped that computers would play a major role in student learning, their major benefit was as a link between all members of the New Pathway community. The computer also offered us a medical literature search service, heavily relied upon by all the students, and some teaching programs, most of which were in the developmental stage during our first two years in the new curriculum. Attempts to use these teaching programs as a core component of the New Pathway curriculum were doomed to failure because of lack of program software. We learned how to use word processing and literature search services, but we were unable to use computers as an integral part of medical education.

The Patient–Doctor Curriculum

The clearest example of the supposed softness of the New Pathway project was the Patient–Doctor course, which sought to offer students early clinical experience and exposure to the humanistic aspects of medicine—sociology, psychology, anthropology, medical ethics, and other related areas. Although most students found the early clinical experience one of the greatest assets of the New Pathway project, the remainder of the curriculum had equal numbers of supporters and critics.

The clinical experience offered by the Patient–Doctor course literally began during the first week of medical school. As we studied each part of the body in anatomy, we also began learning the physical examination of that portion of the body. At the same time, we were developing interviewing and history-taking skills. Although critics of this approach point out that early first-year students lack the knowledge necessary for taking medical histories and performing physical examinations, such critics miss the point of these early experiences. When we were taking a history we were not eliciting all of the pertinent information related to a patient's complaints; rather, we were beginning to learn important skills: talking with patients and touching them. As our medical knowledge grew, so did our history-taking and physical examination skills. By the end of our second year, as we prepared for our clinical rotations, we had been interviewing and examining patients for two years. Walking into a patient's room no longer elicited fear. Asking a patient to undress or performing a pelvic or rectal examination did not inspire terror. Talking with patients about their sexual history or about alcohol and drug abuse was familiar territory. While many of the New Pathway students felt that a more extensive clinical experience before starting clerkships would have been beneficial, none questioned the advantages of starting to interact with patients early in their medical school experience.

Another advantage of this early clinical exposure was of a more emotional nature. The first two years of medical school can be discouraging. Many students enter medicine because they want to be clinical practitioners, yet in a traditional curriculum their first interaction with patients does not occur until late in the second year. They spend the first year and a half in the classroom, a situation not unlike their previous four years of college. The New Pathway project gave us an early taste of what we all wanted. We learned how to talk with patients, how to use a stethoscope, and how to examine the abdomen. After each clinical session, it was somehow easier and more exciting to return to our rigorous study of the basic sciences, having been made aware once again of the important relationship between the basic and the clinical sciences.

These clinical sessions were only a small component of the Patient–Doctor curriculum. Most of the course served as an introduction to psychology, anthropology, sociology, public health, medical economics, and other paramedical fields. The course was built around a weekly lecture and a weekly tutorial session, both of which had associated articles, book chapters, or other assignments to be completed beforehand. Although many of the readings, lectures, and tutorials were valuable, most students found them an unnecessary distraction from their basic science work and other electives. A major reason for this dissatisfaction was the way the Patient–Doctor course was sited in the curriculum as a whole; instead of being a self-contained block, it spanned all four years. Feeling overwhelmed by the basic science tutorials, cases, laboratories, and lectures, plus the required electives, most students paid less attention and gave less time to the Patient–Doctor curriculum. On the other hand, some students found this part of the New Pathway project the most intellectually stimulating of their first two years. Ultimately, apart from the clinical sessions, the Patient–Doctor course must be judged one of the less appreciated aspects of the New Pathway curriculum, given the amount of time devoted to it.

The fact that it was not always well liked, however, does not mean that the Patient–Doctor curriculum did not achieve its goals. As in much of medical education, some learning occurred by osmosis. The designers of the curriculum had virtually assured that students would learn something by simply devoting seven or eight hours a week to the subject. More significantly, they sent a message to the students that the issues involved were important in a general medical education. So although many of us questioned why we spent an hour a week in the Patient–Doctor lecture, no one questioned the importance of cultural issues in clinical medicine, the value of decision trees in helping clinicians, or the necessity of physicians' understanding epidemiologic principles. At the end of four years, despite our nagging and complaining, we had learned a great deal about medical economics, clinical decision-making, anthropology, psychology, medical epidemiology, and medical ethics.

At the end of two years, many of the New Pathway designers' objectives had already been met: we were independent learners, we knew how to work with others, we believed in the relationship between the basic and the clinical sciences, we were comfortable with patients, and we had discovered a great deal of information and many facts while becoming cognizant of the limits and uncertainty of medical knowledge. The costs included a fair amount of student anxiety, occasionally difficult conflicts in tutorial groups, and strained relations with the students in the traditional curriculum. Most of us felt that, on balance, we had done fairly well.

The Clinical Years

For the most part, our experiences in the required clinical rotations resembled those of students in the more traditional curriculum: we worked in the same hospitals with the same house officers, attending physicians, and patients. What was different was how the rotations felt to us. Like all medical students, we found the third year new and unfamiliar; but some problems were unique.

Perhaps the greatest change was our removal from the protected, insulated classrooms of the New Pathway project to the large hospitals affiliated with Harvard Medical School. For the first two years we had had our own faculty, our own classrooms, our own administrators, and a generally controlled and isolated environment. In the hospitals the New Pathway project was looked upon only as "some new curriculum," supposedly soft, and many were anxious to prove that it was an inferior approach to medical education. It was not unusual to hear attending physicians and house officers attacking the program, especially in the clinical rotations that differed substantially from the more traditional ones. A few examples will demonstrate what we experienced.

The core medical rotation had a number of innovations. Some worked, and others did not. One innovation backfired in a serious way. In an effort to ease the transition from classroom to ward, the first two weeks of the rotation focused on gradually introducing us to the medical teams. We spent the first part of the morning in conference, after which we joined up with our teams, only to return to our own conferences later in the day. This process did ease our transition, but it also separated us from our teams, so that we never forged the early student–house officer relationships necessary for a well-functioning ward team. The interns and residents resented the fact that we were away in the early morning, and we were never able to become involved in the care of patients, since we were not present during the agenda-setting work rounds.

Other clinical rotations also increased the amount of time we spent away from the ward teams. In neurology we were assigned to a separate teaching team. In surgery we spent more time with attending physicians and much less with the house staff in an effort to increase the involvement of senior faculty in the education of medical students. In fact the attempts to increase student–faculty time over student–house staff time and to increase the time spent in the ambulatory setting in each rotation (in addition to the required ambulatory care rotation) were as a whole unsuccessful.

This is not to say that, from the student perspective, all the innovations of the clinical years failed. Almost all of us found the ambulatory care rotation invaluable, both in its pairing of medical students with attending physicians in the clinic and in the exposure it gave us to outpatient internal medicine, pediatrics, dermatology, gynecology, and orthopedics. Although not every student found the outpatient setting as exciting as the wards, we all recognized the importance of having experience in ambulatory care in medical school, given the increasing proportion of outpatient care in all branches of medicine and the fact that many interesting diseases can no longer be found on the inpatient services. More important, many of us found ambulatory medicine different in many respects from inpatient medicine, requiring different skills and attitudes.

Overall, the way in which we learned and what we learned during our final two years were not so radically different from the traditional curriculum as had been our first two years. Like all other medical students at this stage, we learned from our interactions with the house staff, attending physicians, and patients.

One large difference remained—the continuation of the Patient–

Doctor curriculum. Every Wednesday afternoon we were freed from our ward responsibilities to return to our Patient–Doctor tutorial group, the same one we had been part of during the first two years. On these afternoons we would often discuss our experiences on the wards, usually in a framework provided by the curriculum designers. At other times we had specific reading assignments and discussions on a variety of topics, including interviewing skills, medical economics, health promotion, and disease prevention. Our absence from the rotations on these afternoons undoubtedly alienated us from the house staff, but many of us found it to be worth the inconvenience. The Patient–Doctor course gave us a chance to reflect on what it was like finally to be taking care of patients. More than just a psychotherapy group, the course offered us a safe atmosphere in which to share our experiences, feelings, fears, and hopes. Each tutorial group was different; some melded better than others, but virtually all of us found our third-year experience in the Patient–Doctor tutorial an emotionally and developmentally important one during this year of transformation. Such reflection may have helped us to avoid much of the desensitization that afflicts so many medical students during the demanding third and fourth years.

All that remained of the New Pathway requirements was the completion of the third- and fourth-year basic science requirement and the required thesis. The basic science requirement was fulfilled in many ways. Some students spent time in basic science laboratories, while others took courses at the medical school. Similarly, the thesis requirement was realized in a variety of ways. While some students organized research done during the previous four years, others did original research solely for the thesis requirement. The areas of investigation varied from red cell proteins to aspects of medical education. Many students found these final two hurdles of the New Pathway project to be an inconvenience, but most felt that they had profited from their completion.

Advising and Evaluation

One of the original goals outlined by the designers of the New Pathway project was to improve student counseling and evaluation. In terms of advising, the New Pathway project was programmatically a failure but practically a success. Although virtually all of us developed good relationships with the faculty advisers assigned to us, the New Pathway project failed to inform them adequately about the required and elective details of the new curriculum. Aside from serving as sounding boards for ideas, the advisers ended up learning more about the curriculum from their advisees than the other way around. Fortunately the curriculum designers and administrators were willing to meet with students individually to offer advice, provide information about the curriculum, and help in any other way they could. We also garnered informal advice from faculty with whom we had forged close relationships.

Another goal of the New Pathway project was to improve the process of feedback to students regarding their performance. Timely and constructive feedback is rare to nonexistent in most medical schools. To many faculty, feedback means a grade. The New Pathway project begged to differ and made strides to improve both student evaluation and feedback on performance. Most of the changes were effective.

In terms of student evaluation, one important change was the decision that all grades would be pass or fail, without further characterization in terms of grade. Each grade, however, was supplemented by a written statement, detailing for each course the student's performance in relating to other students, in tutorials, on oral and written examinations, and his or her enthusiasm for learning. Halfway through each block the tutor would meet with each student to provide feedback on performance. Such timely feedback gave the student opportunity to act, making improvement more likely. These sessions also gave the student an opportunity to give the tutor feedback, and such was often provided, perhaps surprisingly, given the power of the tutor to grade.

In some instances the means of assessing student performance were completely altered. While some blocks used standard multiple-choice, short-answer, and essay examinations, many curricular blocks instituted the so-called Triple Jump, an exercise of three parts. In the first, under examination conditions students would read a case and be asked a number of questions about the case in written format. Such questions stressed hypothesis generation over factual knowledge and asked students to give their thoughts on the case and a description of how they would go about better understanding the case.

In the second part of the Triple Jump, students would have the rest of the day and night to research the issues related to the case. This could include reading textbooks, tracking down journal articles, consulting expert resources (as long as we told the expert that we were under test-taking conditions and showed them the written case). The only people we could not talk to were other students in the New Pathway project. Our research was focused on part three of the Triple Jump.

The last part of the Triple Jump was an oral examination given by one or two expert examiners. Sometimes these were faculty members in the New Pathway project; at other times they were guest experts who were unaffiliated with the program. On occasion under rather stressful conditions, students were asked to give a brief formulation of the case, to outline what they had done to research it, and to state their conclusions, including a diagnosis. That was the easy part. During the rest of the session the examiner probed the student's breadth and depth of knowledge in the subject areas related to the case, always involving the major areas covered during that course. Questions ranged from the general conceptual to the specific factual. Many students in the traditional curriculum regarded the Triple Jump as something of a joke, but in many ways it was the most difficult examination possible. Examiners would frequently question with the purpose of finding the limits of our knowledge, only then to start questioning in a different area, again getting more detailed until we could not answer.

Besides being a challenge, this kind of test was also an intense and valuable learning exercise, often used by course designers to cover subjects that had not been dealt with during the course. It always involved a totally new case, often concerning a subject or concept that we had not encountered. For example, during the Identity, Microbes, and Defense course, which covered the subject areas of pathology, immunology, and microbiology, the case was viral hepatitis, an area we had touched upon only briefly. The oral examination tested our knowledge of the hepatitis virus, mechanisms of cellular damage and neoplasia, pathology of the liver, the immune response, and the clinical presentation, diagnosis, and treatment of hepatitis. This test exemplified how the New Pathway project changed both what we learned and the way we learned.

Evaluation and feedback in the clinical years remained virtually unchanged from traditional methods. As was typical in the traditional clinical rotations, feedback was scanty and often more critical than constructive. Few rotations gave examinations, and none of these could have been called a learning experience. In the clinical years, attempts to improve student feedback and evaluation, like attempts to change the form and structure of learning, were unsuccessful.

Students as Curricular Designers and Modifiers

Feedback and evaluation should never be a one-way endeavor from faculty to student, and the New Pathway designers and administrators were well aware of this fact. From the very beginning, when the New Pathway project was only an idea, students were actively engaged in designing and modifying the curriculum, and when the New Pathway project was in the planning stages, years before the first group of twenty-four students started, Harvard Medical School students were involved in the process. Some students were asked to join committees formed to explore various aspects of designing a new curriculum, while others sat through experimental courses and tutorials before the first group of students enrolled in the new curriculum came to medical school. Such student involvement expanded when the New Pathway project actually began.

At the start of each course, the course director would talk to the students about the importance of feedback and how we could effect change if we thought there were problems. Each course had a weekly feedback lunch at which problems were discussed among students, faculty, and administrators. More often than not, suggestions regarding basic science courses would show up as changes within the next week or two.

Students were deeply involved in course design in another important way: all the curricular design groups had student members, as did the Steering Committee. In these forums, too, student concerns and suggestions could influence course design, if not immediately, then the following year.

Summary

The first four years of the New Pathway experiment had many positive aspects. There seems little question that we had more fun learning than did our traditional curriculum colleagues: we were exposed to clinical medicine earlier in our training, we learned through clinical cases, we spent our time problem-solving, we directed the course of our own learning, we worked very closely with faculty members, and we were part of a new and exciting experiment in medical education. In many ways the New Pathway project did prepare us for a lifetime of learning: it constantly reminded us of the limits of our own knowledge, taught us how to expand that knowledge on our own and with the help of others, and forced us to become familiar with the uncertainty that is such a large part of medicine. By closely relating the basic and clinical sciences, the New Pathway project also prepared us for the closer relationship that will inevitably be forged between these two interdependent areas of modern medicine.

Of course the first cohort did not consider the New Pathway project an unadulterated success. One of the costs was a strained relationship between the New Pathway students and their traditional curriculum counterparts. The computers, by no means the essence of the new curriculum, were one of several sources of friction between students in the New Pathway and in the traditional curriculum. From the beginning of the first year, the New Pathway students were distinct from the other 140 students in the class. Although many of us formed close friendships with students in the traditional curriculum, we always felt very separate. This sense of separateness was one of the unfortunate aspects of the New Pathway experiment. Although the inevitable mixing of all students during the clinical years helped to remedy the situation, the separation led to bad-mouthing, rumors, and bad feelings. Whether it was the computers, the weekly New Pathway "Happy Hours," or the money and favoritism felt to be directed our way, many students in the traditional curriculum felt shortchanged and often let their feelings be known. This is not to say the traditional students wished they were New Pathway students. To them parts of the program seemed too soft.

Another cost, perhaps the highest of the new curriculum, was the student anxiety engendered by a new and student-directed curriculum. The New Pathway project moved toward a new kind of learning, one dependent on students, both as individuals and as groups. With sixteen years of traditional learning styles under our belts, we had proved ourselves successful in traditional learning situations; yet we were now faced with an entirely new learning environment, one in which cooperation and self-direction were valued more than individual achievement and simply following the direction of others.

Other failures at the beginning were less important from the student perspective. One of these was the attempt to rely more heavily on computers in medical education. Although the electronic mail system improved communication among students, faculty, and administrators and many students used the medical literature search service, computers by no means revolutionized our learning experience. Given that computers will certainly be important tools in medicine in the future, this shortcoming was unfortunate.

The last failure concerned the attempt to change learning in the clinical years—and perhaps it was not a failure at all. In general the third and fourth years turned out to be little different from the traditional clinical rotations common in medical schools throughout the United States. There were some changes: a thesis requirement, a basic science requirement, a new ambulatory care rotation, and efforts to begin a new rotation combining obstetrics-gynecology and pediatrics. The failure to effect major changes reflects the approach to clinical teaching in the hospitals with which the medical school is associated. As they try to improve learning in the clinical years, educators will have to address more rigorously the realities of life on the wards.

Notwithstanding these shortcomings, from the student perspective many of the changes implemented by the New Pathway project were resounding successes. At the end of medical school most of us departed happy about our decision to be the first group of guinea pigs. We had achieved some important goals: we had learned how to learn on our own and in groups and with little guidance from our teachers; we had learned how to acquire and use medical information; we had come to understand that knowledge does not mean certainty and that medicine is filled with uncertainty; we had been exposed to many paramedical subject areas; we had experienced traditional clinical medicine with increased experience in the outpatient setting; we had each written a thesis, demonstrating expertise in a field related to medicine. Perhaps most important, we enjoyed ourselves while achieving all these goals.

10

Transitional Organization

S. James Adelstein
with Susan T. Carver, Harvey Goldman,
and Myra B. Ramos

In the fall of 1985 executive faculty in the basic sciences discussed how the New Pathway project would relate to educational programs for the other medical students but reached no conclusions. Some departments felt unable to continue supporting two tracks (in reality, three, including the Division of Health Sciences and Technology). Others wanted to continue instruction along strict disciplinary lines. Most departments had a wait-and-see attitude.

Meanwhile, despite some opposition the Faculty Council had approved increasing the number of first-year students in the new curriculum in 1986 from twenty-four to forty, both to meet the requests of matriculating students for more New Pathway slots and to provide a more adequate statistical sampling for purposes of evaluation. What happened next was somewhat unexpected.

In the fall of 1986, after the second cohort of New Pathway students had started the Human Body course, Elizabeth Hay, the head of the Department of Anatomy and Cellular Biology, members of which had served as leaders of both the course and the Oliver Wendell Holmes Society, announced to the other basic science department heads that her faculty had demanded that all students (except those in the Division of Health Sciences and Technology) take the Holmes Society Human Body block in the 1987–88 academic year, both because they were unable to deliver two courses and because they believed the New Pathway block to be a superior means of teaching microscopic and gross anatomy. She asked her colleagues to support changes in the academic schedule so that the Human Body block could be given to all first-year medical students in the initial eight weeks of the year. In presenting the request to successive meetings of the Curriculum Committee and the Faculty Council, Dr. Hay made it clear that aligning the first-year academic schedule with that of the Holmes Society would permit departments to choose whether to continue the traditional format for their courses, to convert to the New Pathway style, or to collaborate with the Holmes Society to formulate a new version. The proposal generated considerable discussion and some opposition. Specific objections focused on the loss of January and June as separate periods in which to pursue elective courses, research, and travel and the unclear place of pharmacology in the New Pathway curriculum. The general opposition stemmed from a sense that the move would lead irretrievably toward general adoption of the New Pathway curriculum before there had been sufficient experience for a valid evaluation of the program. Nevertheless both the Curriculum Committee and the Faculty Council approved the proposal, instructing the chairman of the Curriculum Committee and the Dean's Office to prepare a schedule and to work with the departments to see how they would like to have the material of their disciplines presented to the class entering in the fall of 1987.

Combined Curricular Design Groups

In December 1986 the Curriculum Committee approved an academic schedule for the first year and part of the second that would include all the customary preclinical subjects. With regard to the New Pathway curriculum the following schedule has remained essentially stable ever since:

No. of weeks	New Pathway	Traditional Pathway
Year I		
8	The Human Body	Cell Biology
		Gross Anatomy
		Histology
		Radiology
10	Metabolism and Function of Human Organ Systems	Physiology
		Biochemistry
		Biophysics

(continued)

No. of weeks	New Pathway	Traditional Pathway
6	Life Cycle I (Genetics, Embryology, and Reproduction)	Genetics Embryology Reproductive Biology
10	Identity, Microbes, and Defense	Microbiology Pathology Immunology Pharmacology
Year II		
10	Human Nervous System and Behavior	Neurobiology Neuroanatomy Neuropathology

During the remainder of the second year students in the traditional curriculum would study pathophysiology and Introduction to Clinical Medicine, while Holmes Society students would study Human Systems, Life Cycle II (adolescence, the middle years, and old age), and physical diagnosis, which was incorporated into the first two years of the Patient–Doctor course.

To explore possible consolidations of the standard and New Pathway curriculums in the various blocks, combined curricular design groups staffed by faculty in the relevant disciplines and by professional educators were established in January and February 1987. The dean asked all these groups to determine the feasibility of providing a common course for all students based upon New Pathway motifs, namely, "the acquisition of skills and attitudes as well as knowledge, a definition of core materials that all physicians should share, utilization of learning methods that are active with less emphasis on lectures to convey information, and the use of case-based and problem-based tutorials that encourage students to direct their own learning." In general, formal instruction was to be confined to mornings, with afternoons left free for self-study and electives. Each group was to determine by March 15 whether a common course of study was desirable and feasible and, if so, to prepare by May 15 a detailed outline and list of course organizers to present to the Curriculum Committee and the Faculty Council. As outlined above, all the blocks were consolidated and approved by the faculty for implementation beginning in September 1987.

The curricular design groups were crucial in fashioning the individual blocks of the New Pathway project. The collaborative efforts of faculty from different departments provided incentive for creating common courses even in departments that had initially shown little enthusiasm. These curricular design groups, now organized somewhat differently, continue to play a central role in curricular development and implementation.

Formation of Additional Societies

With the launching of the Oliver Wendell Holmes Society as a demonstration project in 1984, the Planning Committee was converted, with slightly different composition, into the Steering Committee. This group concerned itself with both short-term and long-term issues. The former were related chiefly to getting the Oliver Wendell Holmes Society up and running; the latter concerned the principles of evolution should the demonstration project prove itself, as all members of the Steering Committee assumed it would. Of the several options conceivable, the committee could envision some expansion of the new curriculum but foresaw the necessity of creating additional societies were the whole class to be involved. Thus in the summer of 1985, even before the first Holmes Society class had matriculated, the committee outlined the attributes of the several societies that might in time be responsible for general medical education at Harvard. A society was to be composed of fellows from the various disciplines of the medical school and about forty students from each class. Each would be responsible for teaching a core of agreed-upon material in accordance with New Pathway pedagogical methods, and each might develop its own elective repertoire.

At the educational workshop in May 1986 Dean Tosteson proposed creating several faculty–student entities called academic societies, each with a master and fellows drawn from all departments who would serve as its faculty and be directly responsible for the general medical education of its students. He believed such entities were necessary because of the marginal time and attention given to medical student education by most faculty members and because of the high degree of fragmentation and specialization in all medical schools. The societies would operate within educational guidelines, to be determined by the faculty, that reflected the pedagogical philosophy of the New Pathway. In March 1987 the Dean convened a task force to address formally the creation of multiple societies. The task force was chaired by Thomas W. Smith, a graduate of Harvard Medical School and professor of cardiology who chaired the Curriculum Committee. He was joined by a distinguished group of senior faculty, most of whom had not actively participated in the New Pathway deliberations, and so brought new perspectives to the proposition. At the educational workshop in May 1987 the task force presented an interim report endorsing the concept of establishing five academic societies (including the Holmes Society) "to assume a principal role in general medical education at Harvard Medical School." The task force suggested that the shared curriculum be designed by the senior fellows according to a matrix concept (discussed below); electives would continue to be available through the departments.

The report offered additional recommendations on the form and function of the societies. The societies should adopt a common calendar with similar shared courses at the outset and common instruments of evaluation. There should be no differentiation of societies by career interest, although some variation in teaching approaches might develop over time. Masters would be responsible for recruiting senior fellows; overseeing, with the fellows, the longitudinal elements of the curriculum; promoting a sense of community; providing academic counseling; playing some role in the admissions process; maintaining the teaching portfolio of affiliated faculty; selecting winners of society-based teaching awards; encouraging student research; contributing to student evaluations; and providing a mechanism for disciplinary action. The masters should have three-to-five-year terms of appointment and devote a considerable proportion of their time to this role. They should have adequate administrative support. Certain activities—final admissions, financial aid, promotions, and internship counseling—should remain centralized in the Office for Student Affairs.

The report of the task force had a mixed reception at the workshop. Although nearly all participants endorsed the proposed composition of the societies and most of the responsibilities proposed for the masters and societies, there was considerable opposition to giving the societies responsibility for the design and delivery of the curriculum. After considerable discussion, both the workshop and subsequently the Faculty Council endorsed the societal concept, "excluding, at this point, curricular matters." The phrase "at this point" allowed the school to get on with the establishment of three new societies to join Holmes and Health Sciences and Technology. In the summer of 1987 the three additional masters were recruited, all of whom were professors of medicine with fine records as both scholars and educators: Ronald A. Arky, an endocrinologist and chief of medicine at Mount Auburn Hospital; Stephen M. Krane, a rheumatologist and laboratory investigator at Massachusetts General Hospital; and Stephen H. Robinson, a hematologist and associate chief of service at Beth Israel Hospital. They named their respective societies for three former Harvard Medical School greats: Peabody, for Francis Weld Peabody, a pathbreaking clinical investigator and first director of the Thorndike Laboratory (of which Arky was an alumnus); Cannon, for Walter Bradford Cannon, an eminent physiologist; and Castle, for William Bosworth Castle, also a former director of the Thorndike Laboratory and a beloved teacher and hematologist.

The Matrix Concept

In his address to the full Faculty of Medicine on May 27, 1987, in order to press for societal responsibility, Dean Tosteson explained his concept of how the societies would participate in curricular development and design in terms of a two-dimensional matrix: on the horizontal axis are required courses occurring at some point during the four years; on the vertical axis are the societies, with their masters and senior faculty, the matrix intersecting so that each society would have a representative from each of the courses. The societies both facilitate student feedback about courses and allow a relatively small group of faculty members and students to work together through all four years. Figure 10.1 shows this matrix as presented in the task force's report.

The matrix concept is an important ingredient in resolving potential conflict between disciplinary expertise and the development and maintenance of an integrated general course of study for all medical students. It permits highly specialized faculty who are also interested in general medical education to wear two hats. Working in a curricular design group with representatives of other societies (the horizontal element), such faculty can apply their special knowledge; working with other senior fellows of their society (the vertical element), they have the opportunity to look at the educational experience in continuity and as a whole. Thus each senior fellow is invited to be both a generalist and a specialist, thinking of the totality of the educational

	Course Block (examples)	A Society Master	B Society Master	C Society Master	D Society Master
Year I	Human Body Gross Anatomy Histology Radiology Cell Biology	Anatomy Sr. Fellow	Anatomy Sr. Fellow	Anatomy Sr. Fellow	Anatomy Sr. Fellow
	Identity, Microbes, and Defense Immunology Microbiology Pathology	Pathology Sr. Fellow	Immunology Sr. Fellow	Microbiology Sr. Fellow	Microbiology Sr. Fellow
Year II	Human Systems Pathophysiology	Medicine Sr. Fellow	Pathology Sr. Fellow	Obstetrics Sr. Fellow	Pediatrics Sr. Fellow
Years III & IV	Surgery Clerkship	Surgery Sr. Fellow	Surgery Sr. Fellow	Surgery Sr. Fellow	Surgery Sr. Fellow

Figure 10.1 Matrix configuration for interaction of societies and sample courses

experience while contributing in a substantive way to one of the building blocks. This structure permits each society to become a minimedical college with its own dedicated faculty drawn from the various disciplines for the purpose of seeing a group of students through all aspects of a shared curriculum but preserving for the faculty the identity that is so necessary for scholarship and advancement. It also allows for proper and identifiable allocation of resources, through the societies for teaching and through the departments for administrative, clinical, and other scholarly activities.

Administrative Structures

A significant factor in keeping medical student education a principal activity of a medical school and its faculty is a proper administrative apparatus. The joint commitment of the dean of the medical school and the university president is an obvious requirement. The situation was particularly felicitous at Harvard: Daniel Tosteson made medical education an explicit primary goal of his decanal leadership, and President Derek Bok extended significant support, devoting his 1984 annual report to an explication of medical education and stating his intention to work aggressively with the dean in his efforts toward reform.

It is also extremely important that principal associates of the dean, rather than junior or part-time members of the Dean's Office with other principal assignments, help the faculty to catalyze reform and establish sustained administrative support for education. Such senior administrators have an established working relationship with senior faculty and departmental administrators.

Changes in the configuration of administrative support for medical education from the inception of the New Pathway as a project reflect the principal developmental phases of the educational reform. The New Pathway project was administered and supported separately from the mainstream educational apparatus (Figure 10.2; see also Chapter 3). In 1987, when the New Pathway model was extended schoolwide, an office was created to centralize staffing and resources for planning, implementation, and evaluation of the entire program in medical student education (Figure 10.3). And in 1992 the structure was again reorganized to support the strengthened role of the academic societies (Figure 10.4; see also Chapter 12).

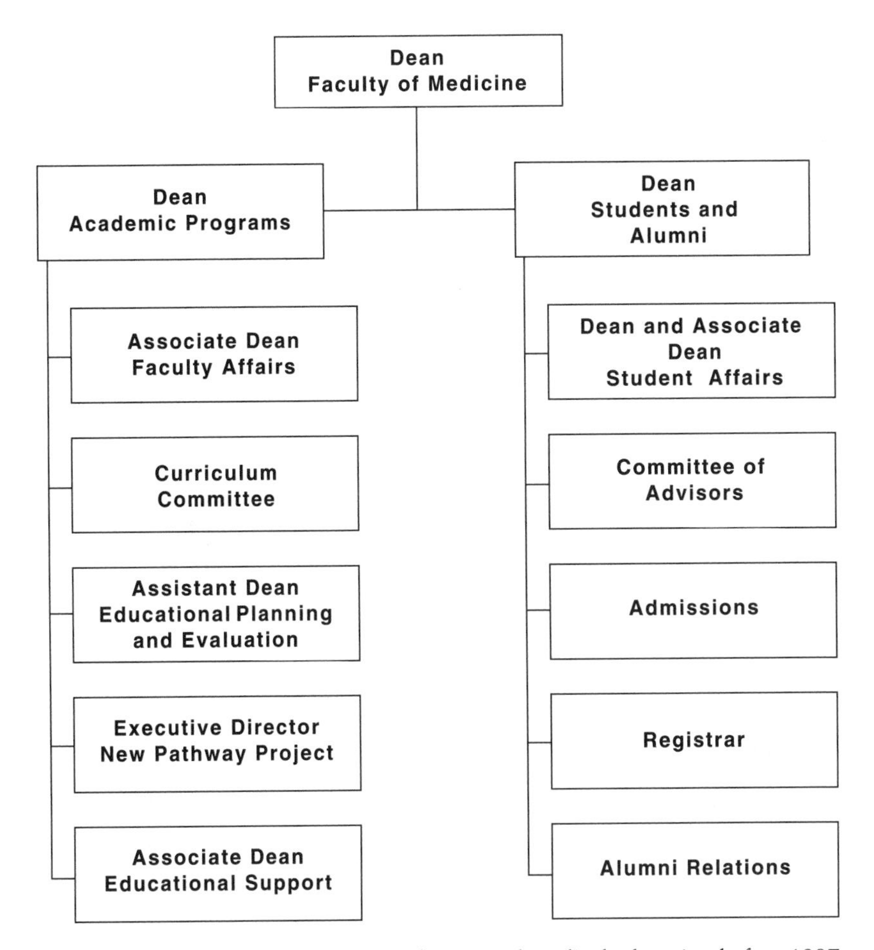

Figure 10.2 Administrative structure for general medical education before 1987

The Curriculum Committee

The crucial part played by the Curriculum Committee in reviewing and approving the New Pathway project was described in Chapter 2. The committee continues to be an important element in educational governance, but its role, size, and composition have all been adapted to changing institutional needs. When it was first established by the faculty, the committee consisted of only ten to fifteen faculty and administrative officers who were involved in major components of the curriculum; there was no apparent need to have representation from

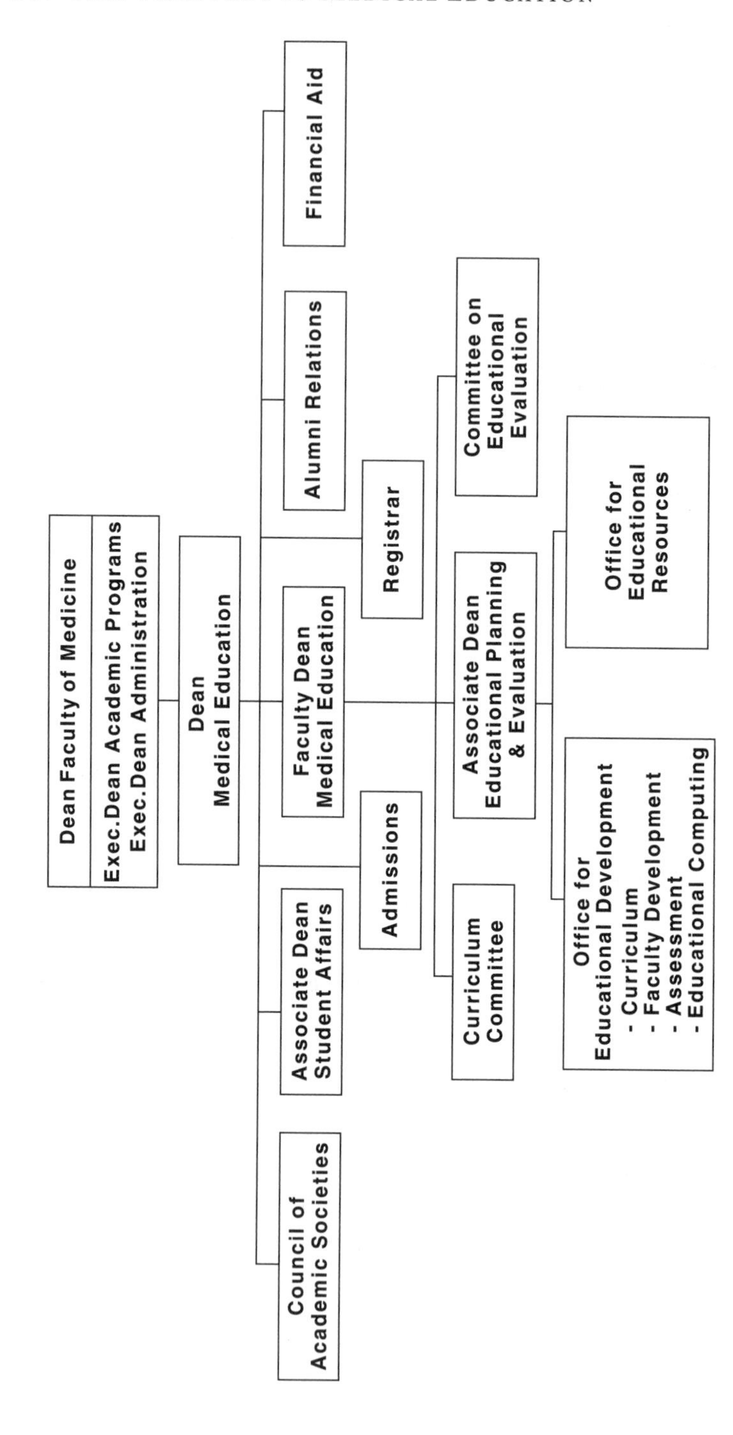

Figure 10.3 Administrative structure for general medical education, 1987

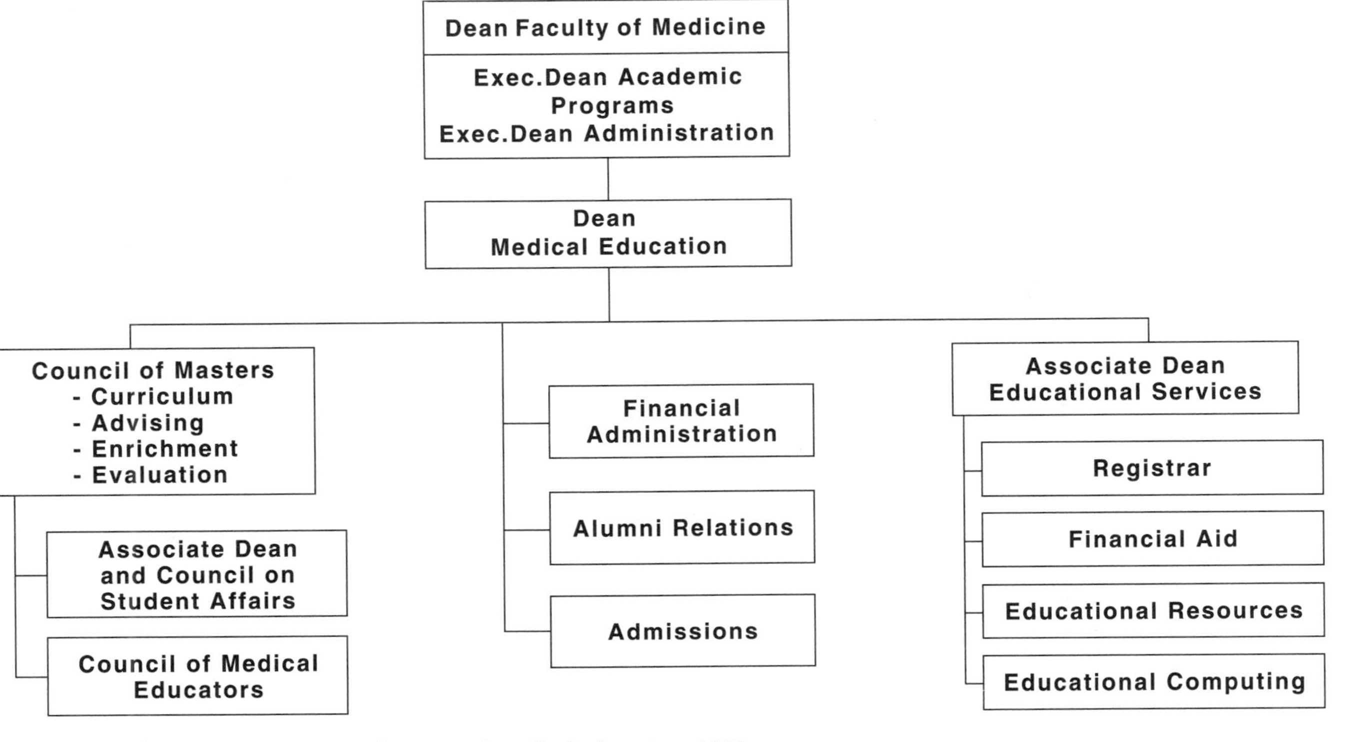

Figure 10.4 Administrative structure for general medical education, 1992

all departments and disciplines. But modifications in the curriculum from 1965 to 1985, resulting in a reduced set of required courses, aroused faculty concerns that the content and identity of the various disciplines might be neglected. To address these issues and to involve students more actively in curricular matters, the Curriculum Committee was enlarged to about seventy-five members. The result was a town-meeting atmosphere that seemed highly democratic but was not always conducive to completing discussions and making final decisions. For some popular issues, such as student grading, visitors would swell the attendance to exceed that noted at the general schoolwide faculty meetings.

Following the decision to extend the New Pathway program to the entire class in 1987, the size of the Curriculum Committee was reduced in recognition of the more extensive use of integrated courses in both the basic and the clinical sciences, which were no longer administered by individual academic departments; the more intimate involvement of the society masters in curricular matters; and the larger roles of the Dean's Office and Office for Educational Development in the administration of the curriculum. In the years 1988–1992 there were about twenty-five members, drawn from the academic societies, other faculty in charge of special components of the curriculum, the deans and other key administrative officers, and students representing all classes. Active participation by faculty from each of the departments and disciplines continued at the level of the individual courses, and close liaison between these courses and the committee was maintained by the use of subcommittees, as described below.

The one standing subcommittee, the Subcommittee on Courses and Credits, reviewed all new courses and assigned credits, subject to final approval by the Curriculum Committee. In addition, there were several subcommittees that dealt with individual required components of the curriculum, including the Human Biology (basic science) courses, the Human Systems (pathophysiology) courses, the Patient–Doctor/Introduction to Clinical Medicine courses, the Social Medicine and Behavioral Science (psychopathology) courses, the clinical courses in the third and fourth years, and the independent project/research requirements. These subcommittees served as coordinating groups and included representatives of the curricular design groups that acted at the level of the individual courses. Each of the subcommittees had representation on and reported to the Curriculum Committee. Additional subcommittees were established as needed to consider other topics such as student grading, uses of computer instruction, and the adviser/mentor system. In general, topics were explored at the subcommittee level and brought to the Curriculum Committee for final discussion and approval if required.

Most curricular issues received final approval by the Curriculum Committee; some more substantive matters, such as major changes in student grading or promotion requirements, went on to the Faculty Council for final decision. The decisions of the Curriculum Committee were implemented by the chair in concert with the relevant group, such as the course directors, the Office for Educational Development, or the Council of Academic Societies.

The functions of the committee included the review of new course proposals by the standing Subcommittee on Courses and Credits, the establishment of the annual school calendar in concert with the Registrar's Office, and the designation of principal faculty leaders such as core course directors and coordinators. The committee considered any other proposed changes involving the students, such as the grading system and requirements for promotion and graduation. It received periodic reports from the various subcommittees dealing with the implementation and progress of the New Pathway components, and considered any proposals for further changes. The composition of the committee and its subcommittees as well as the agendas of the meetings was widely distributed. All meetings were open to faculty and student visitors, and any requests for consideration of items were channeled to the chair.

Student evaluation continues to be initiated by the course directors, monitored by the society masters and advisers, and presented to the Registrar's Office and Promotion Boards for any needed action. A standing faculty committee, the Committee on Educational Evaluation (in 1993 renamed the Academic Societies Committee on Assessment), collects students' evaluations of the faculty and of each required course and conducts detailed reviews of the required clinical clerkships. This information is compiled and sent to the course directors, and summaries of the course evaluations are published annually. The individual faculty evaluations are not published; these are submitted to the course directors for discussion with the individuals themselves. The faculty evaluations are also sent to the relevant department chairman and serve as support for promotion, particularly in the development of the teaching portfolio for the Teacher-Clinician academic ladder (see Chapter 6).

Systematic presentations to the Curriculum Committee of course evaluations collected by the Committee on Educational Evaluation (CEE) began in 1990. In the interim from 1987, society masters conducted intensive course reviews, using input from peer faculty and students, data provided by the CEE, and information collected by an ad hoc course review group. The results were discussed at the Council of Academic Societies, and any recommendations for changes were presented to the Curriculum Committee. This system allowed for an integrated review of courses, involved both basic science and clinical faculty as well as students, and provided comprehensive data for action by the Curriculum Committee.

Office for Educational Development

In 1987 the Office for Educational Development was established to provide to the entire general medical education program the educational expertise and support that had been used in designing and implementing the New Pathway pilot project. This was a major step for a faculty hitherto unused to the participation of professional educators in curricular matters. As noted in Chapter 3, the pilot curriculum for the Oliver Wendell Holmes Society was supported and managed by a core project staff that included experts in curricular and faculty development as well as administrative and support staff. This group worked closely with the relatively small group of faculty members who had signed on to design and teach the innovative program. When the New Pathway curriculum was extended to the entire school, it became essential to reorganize the professional and administrative staff to support the larger goal and to work with the larger number of faculty who would now be involved.

The complex, interdisciplinary design of the basic science blocks and the new teaching methods that emphasized facilitation rather than information transfer constituted unfamiliar demands for those course leaders who had not been involved in the New Pathway pilot program; even for those who had been, the extension of their courses to the entire first-year class involved recruiting and preparing four times the original number of tutors. The New Pathway project staff suddenly found itself coping with several challenges at once: working with much larger numbers of students and faculty, developing productive relationships with faculty who were still traditionally oriented, negotiating and adjusting to the consolidation of two curricular tracks for the class of 1991, and pioneering new clinical clerkships for the Holmes Society classes of 1989 and 1990.

To centralize and simplify the administrative structure supporting medical education, the newly formed Office for Educational Development (OED) merged the New Pathway project staff with several previously separate units and activities: Dean's Office staff working with such faculty groups as the Curriculum Committee and the Committee on Educational Evaluation; and (in 1988) the former Office for Educational Support, which managed educational materials and direct classroom logistic support. The OED consisted of six educators, several part-time faculty members, a full-time student fellow, and twenty-three administrative and support staff.

The two major goals of this unit were to assist the faculty in implementing the new curriculum and to incorporate in all courses the pedagogic methods found useful in the New Pathway approach. Both were addressed by assigning to each unified curricular design group an educator as curriculum coordinator. These individuals served as educational consultants to the curricular design groups, as executive producers of the finely orchestrated new curricular blocks, and as liaisons with all the offices and services involved in implementing the program.

Shifting the Organizational Paradigm

The administrative organization developed during the transitional years 1987–1992 had a number of strengths. First, there was (and still is) a senior member of the Dean's Office (Dean for Medical Education) whose principal undiluted activity was medical education. Second, there was a senior and respected member of the faculty (Faculty Dean for Medical Education) devoting significant time to curricular development, maintenance, and review. We were fortunate in attracting to this position Harvey Goldman, an eminent gastrointestinal pathologist, who had been instrumental in implementing the Health Sciences and Technology curriculum and was acknowledged in the school by students and faculty alike for his teaching abilities and organizational skills. Third, there was a team of professional educators, reporting to both deans, who supported faculty development, curriculum design and implementation, and assessment activities.

That organization, however, lacked several important elements:

- A relatively small group of students and faculty who would dedicate some of their time to examining systematically the course of study leading to the M.D. degree and achieving vertical integration of the curriculum
- A few senior faculty who would dedicate 50 percent of their time to serving as instruments of continuing curricular innovation and sustaining the dynamism of the New Pathway project
- A small group of faculty and staff organized to help groups of students with those extracurricular activities so vital to a complete medical education, namely, academic advising and career counseling, research, and other field opportunities, thereby meeting the demands of a multicultural society on the profession of medicine
- Groups of faculty willing to assess the effectiveness of the educational program from various points of view and to address the continuing issue of evaluating students' performance, for purposes of feedback and of curricular impact, and as a basis for recommendation

To meet these additional needs, in the summer of 1992 the role of the societies was broadened and the responsibilities of their masters increased. These organizational changes are documented in Chapter 12. The OED educators and their vital activities were matrixed to the academic societies, while the educational resource and computing functions were allied with the Offices of the Registrar and Financial Aid to form a new cluster of educational services supporting the strengthened society structure.

Finances

The conceptualization and implementation of the New Pathway pilot project were supported by external funding, as noted in Chapter 2. The initial seed money for planning, $97,000, was provided by the Josiah Macy, Jr., Foundation. Subsequent support came from the American Medical International Foundation, the Arthur Vining Davis Foundations, the Goldsmith Foundation, the Exxon Educational Foundation, Raytheon, the R. H. Macy Foundation, Warren Alpert, and the Higgins Trust. The Hewlett Packard Company contributed $5 million in hardware and software development funds for integration of information technology into the learning environment. A major impetus to the progress of the project was a relatively unrestricted $3 million from the Henry J. Kaiser Family Foundation. This grant convinced many doubting faculty that the project was indeed worthwhile and would move forward.

Recognizing that once the new curriculum was no longer a pilot project, financing would devolve upon the school, Harvard Medical School's financial managers developed a rolling five-year plan that gradually reallocated resources for the education of medical students. Previously there had been no budget line explicitly for medical student education or any data on which to base such a figure; each department had contributed its allotted share of faculty time without central accounting of the costs. Thus it is impossible to answer the recurrent question, "How much more does the New Pathway cost than the traditional curriculum?" The implication is that it must be much more expensive; however, that perception may be based on the experiences of those who teach large classes in other types of professional schools. Medical education has always required, in addition to lectures, extensive interactions between faculty and individual students in laboratories, conferences, and seminars, both in the basic sciences and in clinical subjects.

The extension of the New Pathway project was completed for the class of 1991, which matriculated in 1987. Annual updating of the financial five-year plan has included support of the academic societies, described in Chapter 12, which are currently responsible for the design and implementation of the curriculum. The centralized budget for the curriculum is managed by the Dean for Medical Education, thereby relieving the basic science departments of administrative costs for the support of core preclinical courses. In addition, salary support is provided to the departments for faculty who contribute time in excess of that explicitly expected of all faculty for medical student education.

The following table lists the total annual expenditures for the New Pathway program from 1982 to 1991, from planning phases through pilot project through incorporation of the entire class (with the exception of the Division of Health Sciences and Technology). These figures do not include customary contributions of faculty time.

Year	Expenses ($)	Comments
1982–83	59,700	
1983–84	546,900	
1984–85	1,000,000	
1985–86	2,050,000	Pilot, 24 first-year students
1986–87	2,850,000	38 first-year students
1987–88	2,950,000	All first-year students enter societies
1988–89	3,032,000	First cohort graduates
1989–90	3,340,000	
1990–91	3,500,000	New Pathway program for all four classes

During the planning phase (1982–1985) approximately 65 percent of the budget was spent on curricular development (course objectives, case writing, faculty development, administration, and personnel) and 35 percent on compensation for extraordinary faculty time involved. Grants received to support the effort from 1982 to 1987 totaled $6,506,573 in dollars and equipment, sustaining the dean's commitment not to invade institutional funds to develop the program.

Unlike most medical schools, Harvard receives no income from the clinical practices of its full-time faculty or from the reimbursement of administrative costs for research by faculty based at its affiliated hospitals. The clinical departments, however, have supported their faculty's costs of teaching medical students and residents: in 1988 a faculty committee explicitly stated that receipt of a Harvard Medical School appointment carries with it a baseline obligation to teach predoctoral students, M.D. candidates, or Ph.D. candidates without additional compensation. In 1993 the school began reallocating funds to the clinical departments in order to reflect, in part, their contributions to the education of medical students. This allocation utilizes a new database developed from 1989 to 1991 to track faculty teaching effort by department, by individual, and by course or clerkship. Departments conducting clinical clerkships are reimbursed per student-week of instruction plus an administrative fee. Compensation to clinical departments for participating in preclinical core courses is based on departmental contributed effort.

Applicability to Other Medical Schools

Some medical educators have maintained that only Harvard Medical School's possession of a large faculty permitted the expansion of the

New Pathway program to the entire school. They argue that such an undertaking would not be possible at other medical schools with fewer resources. However, the general elements of the New Pathway program, particularly its use of the active learning process, should be applicable to all medical schools regardless of their size. Indeed, given the staggering expansion of medical science information, it may quickly become the only route for general medical education.

At issue are the number of faculty needed, their commitment of time, and the overall financial support available for the program. The size of tutorial groups need not be restricted to only six to eight students; many faculty are comfortable with twice that number, and similar sessions at business schools have sixty to eighty students.[1] Goals and formats must be adjusted to accommodate a larger number, but there is no need to sacrifice the use of an interactive approach, with students sharing in the responsibility to acquire information. Schools with few faculty should be able to reduce the number of contact hours with students and increase the time allocated for independent study. The use of more interdisciplinary courses would require some rechanneling of funds from the departments to support individual faculty and a professional educational unit.

11

The Medical Education Center

Karla J. Pollick

It was clear from the outset that new teaching facilities would be essential in catalyzing and sustaining the changes in educational content and methods envisioned for the New Pathway project, in particular the use of interactive, small-group learning. It was also important that new facilities reinforce and support Dean Tosteson's vision of academic societies as organizations for faculty and student interaction around the program in medical education. The need to modernize and expand the school's teaching facilities provided the opportunity to incorporate these requirements in the design of new teaching space.

The school's need for new teaching facilities was first discussed at the Harvard Corporation's 1981 summer retreat. Immediately afterward Dean Tosteson appointed an ad hoc faculty committee, including more than a dozen of the school's most active teachers, to evaluate existing teaching space and to make recommendations for improvement. At that time nearly every building on campus contained some teaching space, and some classes were being held at the School of Public Health for lack of sufficient space at the medical school. Of equal concern was the physical age and obsolescence of the existing facilities, in particular those for gross anatomy dissection. It was clear that the existing facilities could not support problem-based learning in small-group settings or the type of self-study and computer-assisted learning envisioned for students in the New Pathway program.

Upon completing its evaluation the committee recommended both a large increase in the amount of space devoted to teaching and the consolidation of teaching space in a central facility. Faculty approval of the plan for the New Pathway project in May 1983 reinforced the need to move ahead with these recommendations.

Planning for the new teaching facility in parallel with designing the new curriculum was onerous but essential in reinforcing the changes introduced by the New Pathway project. Construction of the Medical Education Center provided opportunities to consolidate teaching space in one building, improve teaching support capabilities, enhance the technological capabilities of laboratory and other teaching space, and increase the amount of space devoted to small-group, seminar, and tutorial rooms.

Planning and Program Development

Formal planning for a centralized teaching facility began in 1984. The objective of the planning team, which consisted of faculty, administrative staff, and architectural consultants, was to design a space program sufficiently flexible to accommodate teaching needs well into the next century. Several criteria were identified as paramount: centralization in one facility of all direct instructional space and its related support functions, provision of more small spaces to promote intimate and participatory learning, provision of maximum flexibility to accommodate changing needs, and the greatest possible use of existing facilities to minimize the building of new space. A number of user groups advised the project team on key areas such as laboratories for dissection and physiology, tutorial rooms, and society and social spaces.

First the team prepared a detailed inventory of existing space. It then performed a utilization study to quantify the demand for each type of space and to identify peak demand. This work formed the basis for recommendations on the number and types of rooms that should be provided to meet current needs. The team also visited several other schools with innovative curriculums to gain insight into the linkage between facilities and educational approaches.

With this as a starting point, the team conducted its development of the space plan in parallel with the work of the New Pathway planning committees. Changes in curricular content, teaching methods, and skill-building objectives were assessed in terms of their implications for the types and organization of space required. As time passed, the planning team attended New Pathway lectures and tutorial sessions to gain a better understanding of the space requirements. The most difficult areas to plan were those for computer facilities and teaching laboratories.

The program that resulted from this process described the types of space that would be required, the optimal size for each type of room, and the necessary configuration of interrelated spaces. The planning team also developed initial specifications for the finishes in each type of room, to be used in estimating construction costs.

After evaluating various sites for the proposed facility, the planning team selected one of the school's existing quadrangle buildings, Building E. This choice was influenced by several factors. Most notably, use of an existing building as the basis of the proposed facility minimized the addition of new space to the school's inventory and provided the opportunity to renovate existing space that would otherwise remain a liability for the school's capital program. The plan called for renovation of the existing Building E, a U-shaped structure, and the addition of a new wing that closed the fourth side, creating an open space at the center. The majority of conference and tutorial spaces and the commons area were planned for renovated space so that more-sophisticated spaces, such as the dissection laboratories, skills areas (wet and dry laboratory workstations), case-method room, and computer facilities, could be located in the new addition. Moreover, the Building E site was well integrated into the quadrangle, close to the medical student dormitory, and convenient for students and faculty.

Space Plan

The space plan was guided by the expectation that the new facility would provide sufficient space for the range of New Pathway experiences for the approximately 370 first- and second-year medical and dental students. In keeping with the design of the curriculum, this experience was to include formal lectures, tutorial sessions, laboratory exercises, case discussions, small groups, computer-assisted learning, independent study, and opportunities for informal interaction among faculty and students. Although it was assumed that third- and fourth-year students would spend the majority of their time in the hospitals, the facility would be expected to accommodate a limited number of centrally planned teaching experiences around the clerkships, such as the clerkship in Women's and Children's Health.

Approximately one-quarter of the 27 percent increase in overall teaching space was used for twenty-two new tutorial rooms capable of accommodating twelve to fifteen students around a conference table. On the basis of the experience of the Holmes Society pilot group, it was clear that tutorial groups in the first two years would require a dedicated tutorial room and blackboard so that important elements of discussions could be retained from session to session. To accommodate this requirement, tutorial sessions would have to be scheduled so that a first-year tutorial group would share a dedicated tutorial room with a second-year group. Each room would be equipped with three boards: one each for the first- and second-year groups, and one board for flexible use. The provision of these rooms, equipped to support small-group, interactive teaching, was viewed as the single most important requirement for implementing the New Pathway program.

The plan increased the space devoted to teaching laboratories by almost 30 percent. Dissection laboratories were expanded to accommodate physiology laboratories as well as showers and lockers. Radiology viewing rooms were located adjacent to the dissection laboratories in order to integrate the discipline of radiology with gross anatomy and histology in the teaching of the Human Body course. Other types of teaching laboratories were also targeted for expansion in order to provide greater space for dedicated student workstations and storage, as well as stations for demonstration and discussion. Space devoted to teaching/laboratory support was increased only slightly because centralization was expected to generate efficiencies.

The plan also specified a number of qualitative improvements. Space for storage of equipment, supplies, and audiovisual material as well as for laboratory and computer support was located adjacent to instructional space. A control room was added to permit the remote recording of lectures in the amphitheater and case-method room. Tutorial rooms were to be near teaching laboratories. Careful consideration of interior finishes and special features ensured both the quality and usefulness of the space.

A case-method room was added to the school's inventory of large meeting rooms (with a capacity of 50–100 people) and conference rooms. The room accommodates 80 people and is modeled upon classrooms at the Harvard Graduate School of Business Administration.

The horseshoe-shaped design and tiered seating facilitate interaction within a larger group. The room has proved particularly useful for clinical presentations, faculty development conferences, and student–faculty meetings. It was expected that the addition of seminar rooms specifically for medical-student teaching would relieve some of the severe scheduling pressures on the school's meeting rooms.

Design Development

On the basis of their work in developing the space program as well as their initial thinking about the design, Ellenzweig Associates, Inc., was selected in late 1984 to design the Medical Education Center. Working closely with the planning team and faculty involved in the New Pathway project, the architects incorporated the requirements articulated in the space definition program into a vibrant and innovative facility that promoted the objectives of the New Pathway.

The success of the design can be attributed to several themes stressed doggedly by the architects in working with the planning team. Chief among these was the nature and types of interactions envisioned for the new curriculum and the society structure. The architects pressed the planning team and deans to abandon conventional wisdom about how traditional spaces such as laboratories and dissection areas should be organized and outfitted and urged them instead to think expansively about the range of interactions envisioned and the relationships between activities and spaces. Planners were encouraged to identify opportunities for designing spaces for multiple purposes.

The design that emerged from these discussions was both innovative and highly functional in terms of supporting the New Pathway curriculum, and in particular small-group, interactive learning. The design also reinforced the identity of the academic societies by using the society structure as a way of organizing teaching laboratories, tutorial rooms, and student–faculty cluster space in the new facility. It gave each society a physical as well as a programmatic identity.

The Medical Education Center is organized around a three-story atrium, which has become the center of informal interaction among students and faculty (Figure 11.1). Immediately adjacent to the atrium is a large amphitheater with the society cluster areas extending around the periphery. The society cluster areas include small lounge areas for informal interaction, student study space (including computer work-

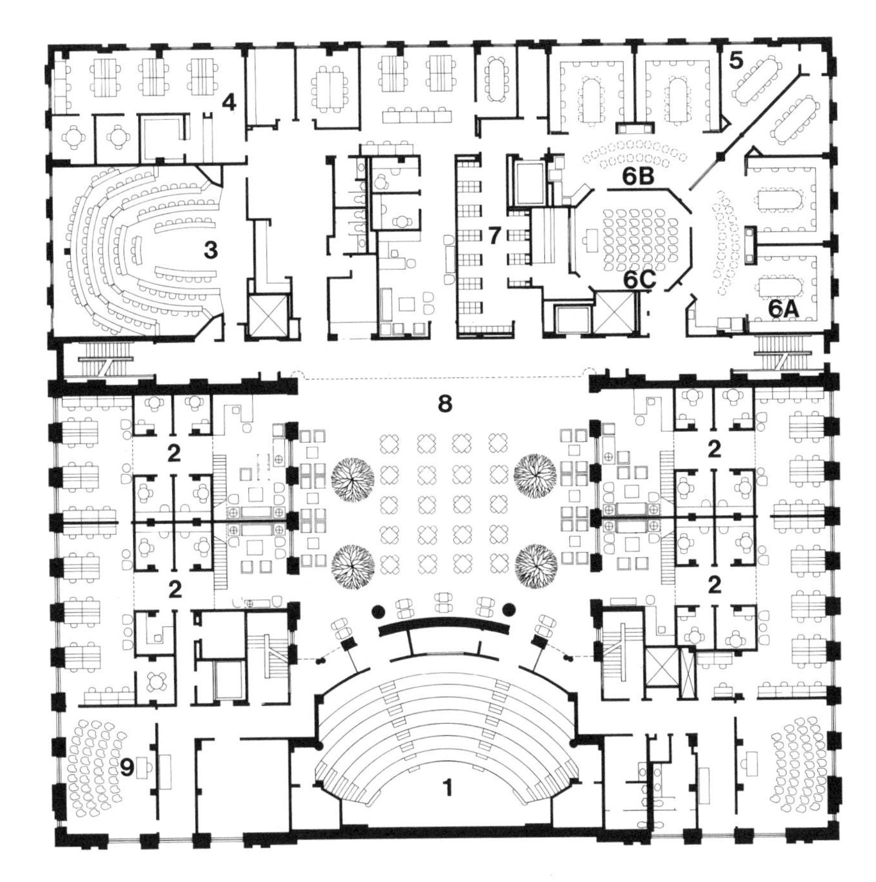

Figure 11.1 Second-floor plan of the Medical Education Center

1 Amphitheater (seating: 214). For full class lectures and demonstrations.
2 Society Cluster Areas. Meeting and study area where students and faculty congregate informally.
3 Case-Method Room (seating: 80). For clinical case presentations and large group discussions.
4 Student Computing Center (seating: 22). Banks of networked computers providing access to educational, commercial, and communications software.
5 Tutorial Rooms (seating: 12). For small-group case discussions.
6A Skills Area Lab Bay (seating: 10). Dry/wet lab bench area.
6B Skills Area Cluster Space (seating: 20). For small-group lab discussions.
6C Skills Area Classroom (seating: 40). For society conferences and demonstrations.
7 Student lockers.
8 Atrium. Student meeting and function area.
9 Program in Medical Education administrative office.

stations), and flexible office space for the master, senior fellows, and society staff.

Dedicated skills areas for each of the five academic societies are located on the first, second, and third floors of the new wing of the teaching facility. The specifications and requirements of existing teaching/laboratory space were incorporated in the design of the skills areas. Each includes four ten-person laboratory bays with individual workstations and microscope storage. The workstations provide space and equipment for a range of laboratory experiences and accommodate the use of microscopes at every seat. Each student is assigned a laboratory locker and work area that he or she keeps for the first two years.

Each of the skills areas has five dedicated tutorial rooms corresponding to the assignment of tutorial groups by society. In addition, each skills area has a dedicated forty-person classroom for larger breakout discussions of the laboratory experience. The layout of the skills areas also allows groups of twenty to work at either end of the room. The rooms are equipped with television microscopes and radiology viewboxes to encourage this type of small-group discussion.

An important feature of the Medical Education Center is a suite of examination rooms to facilitate the teaching and evaluation of clinical skills. The suite was added as a means of facilitating the teaching of clinical skills together with the basic sciences in the first two years of medical school. The rooms are equipped with one-way glass and videotaping capabilities and are used for live observation of students interviewing and examining standardized patients. Students in the Patient–Doctor courses use the rooms for practicing physical examination techniques and interviewing.

Project Cost and Schedule

The total cost for the project was approximately $25 million. Of this total, $12 million was spent on renovation of existing facilities and $13 million on new construction. Some of the costs associated with renovation included the cost of renovating space for those displaced by the project as well as the cost of upgrading a select set of decentralized facilities (an amphitheater and program administration space).

The construction schedule for the Medical Education Center was driven to a major extent by the need for space to accommodate the extension of the New Pathway to the entire school. Preparation of detailed design and construction documents took approximately one year. Renovations required for relocation of the building's existing occupants were done concurrently in order to prepare the site for construction. The new construction began in August 1985 and took approximately twenty months. Renovation of the existing Building E structure got underway in the spring of 1986 and was completed by September 1987.

Lessons to Date

The Medical Education Center supports the evolving needs of the teaching program and continues to generate a sense of synergy around medical education. Twenty-four-hour access encourages students to use the building for interaction with classmates and faculty and for private independent study in society study rooms, tutorial rooms, and skills areas.

The most successful spaces have been the atrium, case-method room, dissection areas, and tutorial rooms. Since 1990 radiology viewboxes have been installed in all tutorial rooms because of high utilization of X-ray films in the teaching cases. However, owing to increased demand (primarily from elective courses), the introduction of advanced basic science courses for fourth-year students, and the adoption of New Pathway teaching methods by the graduate student program, we found that we had provided too few intermediate-sized classrooms (with a capacity of thirty people). Accordingly, in 1988 we converted several storage spaces to classrooms. By resequencing laboratory courses to maximize use of newer laboratory facilities and converting older teaching labs to classrooms, we added two thirty-person classrooms in 1993 and are planning to add four more in 1994.

Besides adding several new classrooms, we are enlarging the classrooms adjacent to the skills areas. These rooms, originally designed to accommodate forty students, are not large enough to accommodate many society-based teaching activities that have attracted additional students. We enlarged one classroom in 1993 and plan to do the other four in future years.

Our experience with the dedicated radiology viewing rooms adjacent to the dissection laboratories has been mixed. The optimal size for this type of teaching is ten to twelve students, but it has been difficult to find enough space and instructors to divide a class of 160 into groups this small. We have had to compromise, dividing classes into groups of sixteen, which is the maximum number that can comfortably fit around a single viewbox for teaching. Many of our radiology viewing rooms are too small to accommodate this number of students. Fortunately, alternative rooms have been found, and the smaller radiology rooms have served other purposes.

The society suites were renovated in 1992 to enhance the function of the societies as faculty organizations for designing and implementing the program in medical education. At least one office was added in each society, and existing offices were reconfigured to include dedicated offices for the master, associate master, senior fellows, and society staff. The society suites have also been equipped to encourage multiple uses (meeting and work space, student study space) and flexibility over time. Computers in the society carrel areas continue to attract students from all four years and serve as an important link with third- and fourth-year students in clinical training. Our experience demonstrates the importance of keeping the society space as flexible as possible in order to accommodate future refinements.

12

Academic Societies

Daniel D. Federman
with Harvey Goldman,
Daniel A. Goodenough, and Myra B. Ramos

Before 1987 the only enduring student organizations at Harvard Medical School were an elected Student Council and various small and disparate interest groups and student–faculty committees. To first-year students especially, the faculty of over 3,000 individuals seemed a remote and impenetrable entity. Aside from encounters in individual courses, students rarely met and made friends with faculty members, many of whom lamented the lack of close interaction with the large groups of students who passed through the school.

In 1987 five academic societies were created to provide the framework for students' experience in general medical education. The Harvard–Massachusetts Institute of Technology Division of Health Sciences and Technology is constituted as one of these. The rest of each class is assigned randomly to the Cannon, Castle, Holmes, or Peabody society. Each society is led by a senior faculty member known as a master, who in turn invites additional faculty to share in the society's membership and activities. The societies program is administered by the Council of Masters, which meets twice monthly and is chaired alternately by the Dean of the Faculty of Medicine and the Dean for Medical Education.

Two major faculty roles have evolved. Senior faculty from each basic science course and required clinical clerkship serve as experts on course content, conveying the purposes of the course to the society and the concerns of the society to the course. The same individuals constitute within each society faculty representatives of the entire curriculum (this role is described below).

The other major faculty role is chiefly one of service to the society and its members, providing guidance to students in their decisions about electives, clerkship sequences, joint degree or individual research programs, and, ultimately, careers and internship and residency selection. Several among this group constitute a cabinet for the master, providing a sounding board and dedicated colleagueship in reviews of academic and personal matters affecting members of the society.

Functions

The society fulfills three functions: academic, support, and personal.

The academic functions focus on general medical education. Being drawn from the principal courses, the faculty appreciate all aspects of students' experiences and are able to provide excellent guidance to course planners. On a regular rotation the faculty, medical educators, and students of each society conduct a comprehensive review of each course. Using formal student questionnaire results, faculty reviews of course content, and peer reviews from attendance at lecture or tutorials, the review committee meets with the course directors and curriculum coordinator to understand their intent and to communicate the responses of students and faculty. The master and administrative assistant then prepare a formal report on the course, which is submitted to the Council of Masters and the Curriculum Committee. This continually evolving set of course reviews then becomes the basis for modification of the curriculum and teaching efforts. It also provides a means of integrating the courses over the four years of the curriculum.

The societies provide the organizational framework for the tutorial aspect of the basic science courses. Tutors are invited to concurrent membership in a society and thus have an opportunity to know their students better than was previously possible in the medical school curriculum. At the end of each block the tutor prepares an evaluative summary of the student's performance and, after reviewing it with the student, submits it to the master. The master thus acquires a comprehensive and up-to-date picture of the student's performance on the basis of which to provide guidance and, if necessary, corrective help. Additional academic responsibilities of the societies include supervision of the requirement for advanced work in basic science or a project or thesis. A schoolwide enrichment program provides the framework to help students to identify projects and obtain funding if needed, and to approve proposals developed in conjunction with research advisers in each society.

Medical school is a demanding and stressful experience. Students confront trauma, serious illness, death, family disruption, and many additional burdens. Many students feel the need for peer counseling, a group identity, or a chance to discuss the unfolding complexity of medical training. The societies provide a natural and safe environment for these concerns. Each student is interviewed by the master within two months of starting medical school. This encounter lays the groundwork for continuing interaction—for advice about special research or career options, for letters of recommendation to outside sponsors or agencies, and, in general, for a number of the functions previously performed by the Office for Student Affairs. The societies are also the chief loci for paracurricular functions, including seminars on ethics, careers in medicine, and interprofessional issues (for example, law and medicine, religion and medicine).

Reassessment and Change

The year 1991 marked the graduation of the first class all of whose members had been part of the New Pathway project. This gave us an opportunity to assess the early functioning of the academic societies. They had clearly begun to achieve the rich faculty–student and student–student interaction for which we had hoped, but they had not assumed responsibility for the curriculum or the span of medical education, and they had not involved sufficient faculty to develop curricular innovation. Consequently, we decided to enhance the authority of the masters and to ask them to devote 50 percent of their working time to this role. The new masters were to be distinguished medical scientists or scholars of the rank of a department chair and were to form a council that would be responsible for curriculum, pedagogy, and student affairs. In addition, each master was to assume a policy and supervisory responsibility on behalf of the school as a whole. One would supervise curriculum policy and management; one would oversee admissions and multicultural affairs; one would be responsible for developing new approaches to assessment of students, courses, and program; one would oversee academic enrichment (joint degrees, research, community activities); and one would lead the development of a comprehensive program of advising.

Despite a national search and the identification of excellent potential candidates, it became clear that at this stage of the school's and the program's development, intimate knowledge of the school and the faculty was needed in order to carry out the master's role. The final appointments were therefore made in July 1992 from existing tenured faculty, with careful attention to gender, field of specialization, and personal style. In the event, two professors from basic science departments and three from medicine were chosen and given the unique charge of assuming responsibility for all aspects of undergraduate medical education. The new organizational structure, called the Program in Medical Education, began at this time.

The Council of Masters has charge of the entire budget for medical student education and all faculty compensation for teaching. Reimbursement is made to the department rather than to faculty, and decisions about faculty participation are made jointly by department chairs, course directors, and the masters. The master in charge of the curriculum and the senior educator decide on compensation for faculty who play major teaching roles. Similarly, all the masters have budgets from which to make payments recognizing major faculty service to the societies. The departments retain authority to appoint and promote faculty, but the masters have an important role in evaluating new and continuing candidates for faculty positions.

The masters and the Dean for Medical Education are now responsible for conducting the program of general medical education. They are the nucleus of a small curriculum committee all of whose members are appointed on the basis of their general, not specialty, interests.

Educational and Administrative Support

Staff

When the leadership and responsibilities of the societies were reorganized in 1992, the professional educators in the Office for Educational Development were individually assigned to the societies to support their curricular initiatives and to assist the society faculty in their oversight of the four-year program. These educators also report to the Director for Medical Education and meet as a Council of Medical

Educators to organize joint efforts to benefit all societies. At this time additional staff were provided to each society, including a person to administer both intersociety responsibilities on behalf of the school as a whole (admissions and multicultural affairs, enrichment, advising, assessment, and curriculum) and intrasociety activities.

Educational Assessment

The comparative evaluation of the Oliver Wendell Holmes Society pilot and traditional student cohorts has been described in Chapter 8. In 1991 evaluation was reorganized to embrace a wider spectrum of issues and activities: the assessment of student performance in courses and in special exercises, faculty review of courses and clerkships in collaboration with the Committee on Educational Evaluation, post-course evaluation of courses and teachers, functions of the Promotion and Review Board, and design of a series of measures both to assess the ongoing program and to follow the professional development of graduates.

Educational Research

While developing and mounting the new curriculum, Harvard Medical School educators and faculty have studied the educational process and contributed to the literature in this field. They meet regularly to discuss journal articles, to review research projects in progress, and to hear presentations by visitors.

Curriculum Index

In order to monitor and coordinate content in an interdisciplinary, case-based curriculum such as the New Pathway project, it was necessary to create a computerized curricular indexing system. Using key words, one can ascertain where topics such as diabetes, endocrinology, and ethics are presented at any point in the four years; this knowledge is an invaluable tool in vertical integration efforts.

Educational Services

As mentioned in Chapter 10, certain academic support functions (Educational Resources, Educational Computing) were linked to the

Offices of the Registrar and Financial Aid to form a centralized locus of services supporting the educational experience of students and faculty in the societies. Currently, an integrated student information system that will start its pilot phase in 1995 is being developed to facilitate data sharing among staff offices and to provide students and faculty with direct access to appropriate information.

Educational Resources

This unit works closely with faculty and educators on such curricular implementation matters as acquiring equipment; providing a wide variety of course materials, including microscope slides and X-ray films used to supplement tutorial cases; obtaining textbooks and establishing library reserves; setting up laboratory exercises; providing media support; and coordinating classroom and meeting space needs.

Another important resource is the database on faculty teaching effort (as measured by student contact hours), compiled from information provided by core course and clerkship directors. This database also permits coordination of the recruitment of teachers for the various courses.

Educational Computing

An Educational Services staff manages the acquisition and development of educational courseware in collaboration with medical computing laboratories at Massachusetts General Hospital and Brigham and Women's Hospital, organizes student computing assistants to provide support to student network users, and works to foster an information culture at Harvard Medical School. The recent addition of Internet and Gopher capabilities to the student network has augmented both the possibilities and challenges of accessing and managing medical information (described in Chapter 7).

13

Lessons for the Future

Daniel C. Tosteson
with Harvey Goldman

Designing and implementing the New Pathway has revealed both conceptual and organizational issues that will shape general medical education in the years to come. Conceptually, three broad concerns are particularly significant: the changing nature of information relevant to medical practice and medical science, the resultant need for new ways of thinking about human health and disease in the emerging age of molecular and cellular medicine, and the need for a deeper understanding of the process of learning to learn. At an organizational level, the fundamental question is how to structure faculties of medicine so that they will devote more coherent and creative thought to these difficult conceptual issues.

The most obvious change in information bearing on medicine and medical science is quantitative. Most of the remarkable increase in medical knowledge arises from the invention of new technologies that permit new realms of awareness. The history of biomedical research is a story of our capacity to observe and manipulate smaller and smaller parts of living organisms. Light microscopy revealed cells; electron microscopy visualized organelles and the aggregates of macromolecules that make up membranes and the cytoskeleton; absorption and emission spectroscopy and diffraction of various frequencies of electromagnetic radiation illuminate the locations and properties of atoms in the macromolecules and smaller molecules in the system. In each of these additional rooms in the mansion of life that technology permits us to enter, we see a myriad of new and hitherto unnamed images. In order to think about and communicate these impressions, we invent new words or, more often and confusingly, use old words in new ways. Witness the bewildering array of jargon that permeates the literature of the clinical and basic medical sciences.

The quantity of medical information grows both by probing more deeply into the molecular and cellular mechanisms of disease and by realizing the medical relevance of many fields of inquiry that were previously felt to be quite distant from the bedside, such as statistics, economics, sociology, social anthropology, and ethics. An ever-larger number of fields of learning are now recognized to be components of the necessary foundation for medical practice, and knowledge in each of these fields is becoming deeper and more textured.

The rate of increase of medical information is also accelerating; learning is autocatalytic. Each discovery or invention creates more questions than it answers. The process rather resembles a hypercard. We keep adding new cards that connect the proliferating realms of awareness. Each new card is the base for creation of an additional array of cards. This logarithmic growth of medical information seems likely to continue for the foreseeable future.

Most scientific, including biomedical, knowledge is recorded in words or word equivalents (alphabetic symbols or abbreviations). As the mass of information grows, this linear mode of thinking about, recording, and communicating medical information becomes more ponderous and less effective. The presentation of sequences of bases in the DNA of the most recently cloned genes published weekly in *Nature* or *Science* illustrates the problem vividly: they are often neither useful nor beautiful. We need to learn how to think and communicate about modern human biology in new ways. In order to conceive the functions of the human body in molecular and cellular detail, we will need new languages that make more creative use of the capacity of our visual and auditory systems to integrate complexity.

Given the large number of different kinds of molecules (approximately 10^9) in the human body, distributed in different amounts in approximately 10^{14} cells, all reacting with one another to varying degrees, it seems unlikely that a comprehensive description in terms of atoms will be useful or feasible. The single capital letters used to denote specific amino acids and nucleic acid bases have no formal connection with the alphabet of the periodic table of elements. Though more convenient than an atomic alphabet, such an approach falls far short of the goal of creating a vocabulary and syntax that will describe an organism. For that we require a new form of synthesis of complexity that may look more like graphic art or music, or a combination of both, truly new ways of thinking about the human body as a molecular system.

The advent of molecular medicine, with its breathtaking promise for more specific and timely diagnosis and more powerful, effective, and dangerous treatments, makes the need for a new language of life all the more urgent. Physicians require such a paradigm in order to think about their patients in ways that permit appropriate access to molecular detail when such knowledge is crucial for diagnostic, preventive, or therapeutic action, without the burden of such a ponderous accumulation of facts that it will impede analysis and decision. The use of computers permitting rapid access to and retrieval of such arrays of potentially useful information is one obvious strategy that is already being explored in hospitals and clinics.

In light of the continuously increasing rate of growth of medical information and the wealth, depth, and connectedness of this information, it is becoming progressively clearer that medical education cannot be confined to a limited period at the beginning of a physician's career, but rather must be a continuous, lifelong process. Programs leading to the M.D. degree must have as their principal goal learning to learn. Improving the quality of these programs turns on both a fuller understanding of the mental activity of learning and the reduction of these insights into effective practice.

At a workshop in August 1991 sponsored by the Nordisk Association for Medical Education, participants were asked to describe their most "powerful" learning experiences. Most of the accounts had several features in common.

The most frequently mentioned feature of "powerful" learning was the engagement of the learner's desire and commitment to learn. These feelings usually arose through close personal relationship between student and teacher, between apprentice and mentor. In instances of learning in the clinical setting, the personal relationship was often between doctor as teacher and patient as student.

A second aspect of "powerful" learning is the reinforcement of the desire to learn that comes from success. Even the most ardent minds weaken with recurrent failure. Confidence built on small but steady achievements seems to be an essential ingredient of learning effectively. Usually the learner must believe that it is possible to arrive at or at least to move toward a solution in order to continue working on a difficult problem.

A third element of an effective style of learning is curiosity about relationships between events. This attitude often derives from skepticism or doubt about the currently accepted explanation. Doubt stimulates the creation of fresh hypotheses that invite testing by further observation or experiment. In clinical medicine, curiosity based on doubt is the route toward hitherto unsuspected but more accurate diagnosis. The desire and confidence to learn sustain the courage of the student to take the risk of doubting conventional propositions and creating novel ones.

Fourth and last in this short list of properties of "powerful" learning is the need for repetition. As the old aphorism states, "Practice makes perfect." Desire, confidence, and curiosity come to naught if exercised only once or at long and rare intervals. As with the muscular system, exercise builds strength. All the educational stratagems of schools at all levels may be viewed as devices to entice, cajole, or require students to use their minds repetitively. This imperative persists throughout life. Mental activity seems to follow the rule of evolution: "Use it or lose it."

Most existing programs of general medical education give too little attention to these features of "powerful" learning. Often, teachers are preoccupied with calling to the attention of students bodies of information that the teachers believe are essential or important. The need to structure the learning experiences so that they arouse desire, build confidence, excite curiosity, and reward repetition is usually not near the top of the faculty's list of priorities.

Research is revealing the texture of learning in ways that may prove useful in designing programs of education. I am particularly impressed by the observation of Steven Pinker on the differences between the process that children use in learning the tenses of irregular as compared with regular English verbs.[1] He reports that children master the forms of irregular verbs earlier in life by imitating the sounds made by their teachers (usually parents) and associating the sounds with particular actions. Forms of regular verbs are learned later by grasping a rule (addition of the suffix *–d* or *–ed*). It is not uncommon for children to begin to make errors in infrequently used irregular verbs once they have learned the regular verb rule. These two kinds of learning, associative and rule, apparently are subserved by two different regions in the brain. This hypothesis is supported by the observation that there are partially inherited learning disabilities involving one (rule) but not the other (associative) kind of learning and by reported cases of brain damage by stroke and other insults in which one kind of learning is lost while the other survives intact.

These studies raise the question of whether the structure of experiences designed to promote associative learning may be different from the structure of experiences aimed at deriving and mastering rules. Both approaches are important in learning medicine and the arts and sciences basic to medicine. For example, the kinds of mental work involved in acquiring the names of drugs or even the jargon of specialties such as endocrinology or immunology all fall into the category of associative learning. By contrast, an understanding of the physicochemical mechanism of initiation of the action potential in nerve cells or various types of muscle cells, how these cellular bioelectrical events generate the currents and potential detected in an electrocardiogram or electroencephalogram, the idea of allosterism and its role in regulating the rates of chemical reactions catalyzed by enzymes—all require grasping a number of rules that have been inferred from experiments in physics and chemistry. Greater awareness of these two kinds of learning and better understanding of the most effective ways to promote them could lead to improved design of curriculums for general medical education.

These conceptual issues will be addressed effectively only if faculties of medicine organize themselves to carry out the necessary work. Four aspects of faculty organization for medical education seem to be particularly important. First, the structure should provide incentives for faculty to participate in the design and implementation of the program of medical education. Second, the organization should provide a context within which students can get to know some members of the faculty as persons, outside the narrow confines of the classroom. Third, the arrangements should encourage faculty to consider not only the role of their own specialty disciplines in the curriculum but also the goals and style of the entire program. Fourth, the design should promote continuing assessment of the quality of the educational experience and improvement-seeking exploration.

In most medical schools, academic advancement depends on the quality of research as judged by peers. Criteria for promotion usually list contributions to the design and implementation of educational programs as a minor, albeit positive, term in the equation. Occasionally an excellent performance in the classroom will tip the balance in favor of appointing an individual with a marginal record as an investigator. Most of the time, however, achievements in research outweigh those in teaching, with the result being a gradual devaluation of the importance of teaching in the institution. For education to move up on the list of faculty priorities, it must be recognized as an essential product of the institution, involving the same intensity and creativity of mental effort as research. Indeed, many issues of content and process in educational programs are poorly understood and deserving of investigation. Although such research is pursued in some professional schools, such as the Harvard Graduate School of Business Administration, it is not high on the agenda of most faculties of research universities and certainly of most medical schools. For the priorities to change, academic and financial rewards for teaching and research on educational strategies and tactics must be strengthened. For me, the most important outcome of the New Pathway process at Harvard Medical School has been to increase the attention given by the faculty to the fascinatingly complex and important problem of how to prepare young persons for lifetimes of learning medical practice and science at the turn of the century. Ideally, medical faculties should organize themselves to express the complementarity of educational research and the discovery of new knowledge relevant to the prevention, diagnosis, and treatment of disease.

A second goal of the organization of programs of general medical education should be to encourage close and continuing relations between faculty and students. In many medical schools, encounters between most faculty members and students are brief, oriented to specialized knowledge, and relatively anonymous. Typically these meetings occur in lecture halls during the preclinical years and in the busy environment of the teaching hospital during the clinical years. It is not easy for students to learn enough about individual members of the faculty to become acquainted with different styles of professional living that they might choose to emulate. I mentioned earlier that "powerful" learning often arises out of a strong relationship between student and mentor. It is, of course, impossible to mandate such friendships, but it is feasible to remove obstacles and to make time for them to develop. Similar reflections apply to the educational value of close working relationships among students. Peers promote mutual learning both motivationally and cognitively. Programs of medical education should be organized to take advantage of the powerful effects of mentors and peers on the desire and skill to learn.

The third aspect of organizing general medical education is the need to foster continuity and coherence of the entire *program* and not just the individual component courses. Most faculty members in medical schools contribute to medical education by bringing their special knowledge of some particular segment of medicine or the arts and sciences basic to medicine to the attention of students. The role of that segment in the entire program often receives little consideration. As the mismatch between the amount of information potentially relevant to medical practice and the capacity of individuals to assimilate knowledge grows, the need for informed choices about what to include in the curriculum becomes more difficult and more urgent. These choices should not be made only by specialists isolated from one another but by consensus among a team of faculty who have the responsibility and the authority to design and deliver the entire program. The organization of the program should provide support for nurturing such teams that will draw faculty into the task of creating an ensemble of experiences helpful to students in developing the attitudes, skills, and framework of knowledge necessary to sustain a lifetime of learning in medicine.

The fourth aspect of administering medical education that requires emphasis is providing for continuing exploration of new ways to prepare for the medicine of tomorrow. The content and process of a curriculum leading to the M.D. degree are not a problem to be solved but a set of issues to be worked. This is particularly true at a time when many aspects of the profession are changing at an accelerating rate. Discoveries in the sciences basic to medicine change weekly the ways that doctors think about normal and abnormal functions of the human body. Technology is providing physicians with even more potent, effective, dangerous drugs, devices, and procedures. The practice of medicine becomes progressively constrained by regulations intended to reduce costs but simultaneously to increase access to care for patients who are now underserved. The list of concerns that demand the attention of physicians keeps growing. How to accommodate this deluge of pertinent information in a curriculum of limited duration is an endless task. Faculties should organize for education so that barriers to innovation are minimized. Pilot programs involving some but not all of the class should be encouraged. Mechanisms for assessing outcomes and promoting wider adoption of successful initiatives should be put in place. A spirit of inquiry about the process of learning medicine should be cultivated.

All four of these aspects of faculty organization for general medical education are expressed in the five academic societies that are evolving in the Faculty of Medicine at Harvard Medical School. Implementation of the New Pathway system is still in progress, with societal attention currently focused on the clinical courses and the independent project/research requirements. At the same time, the elements already in place require constant monitoring and refinement to ensure their continued vitality and success. This remains the responsibility of the Council of Masters, the Council of Medical Educators, and the academic societies.

Future efforts must be directed at reducing the number of required courses so that students can individualize their experiences, developing an evaluation system for the program, providing sufficient support and rewards for the faculty, and enhancing the involvement of the academic societies in curricular innovation. As a result of the positive faculty response to the New Pathway approach, it is being extended to postgraduate education in the biomedical and basic sciences at Harvard Medical School and to the Harvard School of Dental Medicine. Two other challenges remain: providing high-quality general medical education in only four years despite the massive expansion in medical knowledge, and exploring the potential for interfacing with the preceding college and subsequent residency years.

Probably the best conclusion we can offer regarding the New Pathway curriculum is to admit that we have not solved all the challenges facing us and do not expect to. We must anticipate continuous adaptation to ever-changing needs in medical information, technology, and society. The promotion of an active system of learning seems like a good beginning.

I hope that the experience of the Harvard University Faculty of

Medicine in grappling with the challenges of general medical education will be useful to colleagues engaged in similar work at other institutions. The perception and formulation of issues and the directions of exploration vary widely among institutions, but we can (and must) learn from one another as we explore how best to prepare physicians to apply the insights of the new biology to the benefit of individuals' health.

Notes

1. Toward a New Medicine

1. A. Kornberg, "Understanding Life as Chemistry," in K. J. Isselbacher, ed., *Medicine, Science, and Society: Symposia Celebrating the Harvard Medical School Bicentennial* (New York: John Wiley and Sons, 1984), pp. 7–17.
2. J. C. Stephens et al., "Mapping the Human Genome: Current Status," *Science* 250 (1990):237–244.
3. R. W. Brimblecombe et al., "Proceedings: The Pharmacology of Cimetidine, a New Histamine H2-Receptor Antagonist," *British Journal of Pharmacology* 53 (1975):435–436.
4. D. W. Cushman and M. A. Ondetti, "History of the Design of Captopril and Related Inhibitors of Angiotensin-Converting Enzyme," *Hypertension* 17 (1991):589–592; M. A. Ondetti, B. Rubin, and D. W. Cushman, "Design of Specific Inhibitors of Angiotensin-Converting Enzyme: New Class of Orally Active Antihypertensive Agents," *Science* 196 (1977):441–444.
5. A. Kleinman, *Patients and Healers in the Context of Culture* (Berkeley: University of California Press, 1980).
6. P. Starr, *The Social Transformation of American Medicine* (New York: Basic Books, 1983).
7. R. R. Edelman, "Magnetic Resonance Imaging of the Nervous System," *Discussions in Neuroscience* 7 (1990):11–63.
8. *Washington Post,* January 29, 1991, p. D1, col. 2.
9. D. C. Tosteson, "Competition, HMOs, Medicine, and Medical Education," in J. I. Hudson and M. Nevins, eds., *HMOs: Academic Medical Centers, Proceedings of a National Conference* (Menlo Park: Henry J. Kaiser Family Foundation, 1981), p. 269.
10. J. E. Murray, J. P. Merrill, and J. H. Harrison, "Renal Homotransplantation in Identical Twins," *Surgical Forum* 6 (1955):432–436.
11. D. C. Tosteson, "Learning in Medicine," *New England Journal of Medicine* 301 (1979):690–694.
12. C. Bernard, *An Introduction to the Study of Experimental Medicine* (1865) (New York: Henry Schuman, 1949), pp. 212–216.

13. H. A. Simon, "A Mechanism for Social Selection and Successful Altruism," *Science* 250 (1990):1665–68.

14. D. A. Schon, *The Reflective Practitioner: How Professionals Think in Action* (London: Temple Smith, 1983).

4. The First Curriculum

1. H. S. Barrows and R. M. Tamblyn, *Problem-Based Learning: An Approach to Medical Education* (New York: Springer-Verlag, 1980).

5. Curriculum Design

1. S. Muller, "Physicians for the Twenty-first Century: Report of the Project Panel on the General Professional Education of the Physician and College Preparation for Medicine," *Journal of Medical Education* 59(11, pt. 2) (1984):1–2.

2. S. H. Kaplan, S. Greenfield, and J. Ware, "Impact of the Doctor-Patient Relationship on the Outcomes of Chronic Disease," in M. Stewart and D. Roter, eds., *Communicating with Medical Patients* (Newbury Park, Calif.: Sage, 1989), pp. 228–245; B. M. Korsch, E. K. Gozzi, and V. Francis, "Gaps in Doctor-Patient Communication. 1. Doctor-Patient Interaction and Patient Satisfaction," *Pediatrics* 42 (1968):855–871; V. Francis, B. M. Korsch, and M. J. Morris, "Gaps in Doctor-Patient Communication: Patients' Response to Medical Advice," *New England Journal of Medicine* 280 (1969):535–540; M. R. DiMatteo and D. D. DiNicola, *Achieving Patient Compliance: The Psychology of the Medical Practitioner's Role* (New York: Pergamon Press, 1982), pp. 55–58.

3. Muller, "Physicians for the Twenty-first Century"; Subcommittee on Evaluation of Humanistic Qualities in the Internist, American Board of Internal Medicine, "Evaluation of Humanistic Qualities in the Internist," *Annals of Internal Medicine* 99 (1983):720–724; American Board of Pediatrics, "Teaching and Evaluation of Interpersonal Skills and Ethical Decision Making in Pediatrics," *Pediatrics* 79 (1987):829–833.

4. D. A. Hamburg, G. R. Elliot, and D. Parron, *Health and Behavior: Frontiers of Research in the Biobehavioral Sciences* (Washington, D.C.: National Academy Press, 1982), pp. 3–21; D. L. Wingard, "The Sex Differential in Morbidity, Mortality, and Lifestyle," *Annual Review of Public Health* 5 (1984):433–458.

5. L. F. Berkman, "Physical Health and the Social Environment: A Social Epidemiological Perspective," in L. Eisenberg and A. Kleinman, eds., *The Relevance of Social Science for Medicine* (Dordrecht: Reidel, 1981), pp. 51–76.

6. H. Weiner, *Psychobiology and Human Disease* (New York: Elsevier North-Holland Press, 1977).

7. T. Mizrahi, *Getting Rid of Patients: Contradictions in the Socialization of Physicians* (New Brunswick, N.J.: Rutgers University Press, 1986).

8. H. Jason, "Evaluation of Basic Science Learning: Implications of and for the 'GAP Report,' " *Journal of Medical Education* 49 (1974):1003–04.

9. Muller, "Physicians for the Twenty-first Century."

10. L. G. Croen, P. D. Lief, and W. H. Frishman, "Integrating Basic Science and Clinical Teaching for Third-Year Medical Students," *Journal of Medical Education* 61 (1986):444–453.

11. V. L. Patel and W. D. Dauphinee, "Return to Basic Sciences after Clinical Experience in Undergraduate Medical Training," *Medical Education* 18 (1984):244–248.

12. V. L. Patel, D. A. Evans, and G. J. Groen, "Reconciling Basic Science in Clinical Reasoning," *Teaching and Learning in Medicine* 1 (1989): 116–121.

13. R. B. Colvin, *Curriculum Guide to Identity, Microbes, and Defense* (Boston: Harvard Medical School, 1990), p. 17.

14. D. E. Melnick, "Development of New Assessment Methods," in K. E. Cotton and J. L. Lawley, eds., *In Service to Medicine* (Philadelphia: National Board of Medical Examiners, 1990), pp. 45–47.

15. A. C. Powles et al., "The 'Triple-Jump' Exercise: Further Studies of an Evaluative Technique," in *Research in Medical Education 1981: Proceedings of the Twentieth Annual Conference* (Washington, D.C.: Association of American Medical Colleges, 1981), pp. 74–79.

16. E. G. Armstrong, "A Hybrid Model of Problem-Based Learning," in D. Boud and G. Feletti, eds., *The Challenge of Problem-Based Learning* (London: Kogan Page, 1991), pp. 137–149.

17. A. Kaufman, "Introduction," in A. Kaufman, ed., *Implementing Problem-Based Medical Education: Lessons from Successful Innovations* (New York: Springer-Verlag, 1985), p. xxii.

6. Faculty Development

1. E. M. Rogers and F. F. Shoemaker, *Communication of Innovations: A Cross-Cultural Approach* (New York: Free Press, 1971); E. M. Rogers, *Diffusion of Innovations,* 3d ed. (New York: Free Press, 1983); R. F. Waugh and K. F. Punch, "Teacher Receptivity to Systemwide Change in the Implementation Stage," *Reviews in Educational Research* 57 (1987):237–254; S. Hollingsworth, "Prior Beliefs and Cognitive Change in Learning to Teach," *American Education Research Journal* 26 (1989):160–189.

2. J. Willems, "Problem-Based (Group) Teaching: A Cognitive Science

Approach to Using Available Knowledge," *Instructional Science* 10 (1981):5–21; R. Glaser, "Education and Thinking: The Role of Knowledge," *American Psychologist* 39 (1984):93–104; G. C. Phye and T. Andre, eds., *Cognitive Classroom Learning: Understanding, Thinking, and Problem Solving* (Boston: Academic Press, 1986); J. S. Brown, A. Collins, and P. Duguid, "Situated Cognition and the Culture of Learning," *Educational Researcher* 18 (1989):32–41; L. B. Resnick, ed., *Knowing, Learning, and Instruction* (Hillsdale, N.J.: Lawrence Erlbaum Associates, 1989).

3. L. Wilkerson and E. M. Hundert, "Becoming a Problem-Based Tutor: Increasing Self-Awareness through Faculty Development," in D. Boud and G. Feletti, eds., *The Challenge of Problem-Based Learning* (London: Kogan Page, 1991), pp. 159–171.

4. H. S. Barrows, *The Tutorial Process* (Springfield: Southern Illinois University School of Medicine, 1988).

5. L. Wilkerson, J. P. Hafler, and P. Liu, "Issues in Problem-Based Learning: A Case Study of Student-Directed Discussion in Four Problem-Based Tutorial Groups, " *Academic Medicine* 66 (suppl.) (1991):S79–S81.

6. H. Jason and J. Westberg, *Teachers and Teaching in U.S. Medical Schools* (Norwalk, Conn.: Appleton-Century-Crofts, 1982); C. B. Meleca, F. T. Schimpfhauser, J. K. Witteman, and L. A. Sachs, "Clinical Instruction in Medicine: A National Survey," *Journal of Medical Education* 58 (1983):395–403.

7. M. A. Smylie, "The Enhancement Function of Staff Development: Organizational and Psychological Antecedents to Individual Teacher Change," *American Educational Research Journal* 25 (1988):1–30; S. W. Bloom, "The Medical School as a Social Organization: The Sources of Resistance to Change," *Medical Education* 23 (1989):228–241; D. A. Goodenough, "Changing Ground: A Medical School Lecturer Turns to Discussion Teaching," in C. R. Christensen, D. A. Garvin, and A. Sweet, eds., *Education for Judgment: The Artistry of Discussion Leadership* (Boston: Harvard Business School Press, 1991), pp. 83–98.

8. M. Silver and L. Wilkerson, "Effects of Tutors with Subject Expertise on the Problem-Based Tutorial Process," *Academic Medicine* 66 (1991): 298–300; C. J. Eagle, P. H. Harasym, and H. Mandin, "Effects of Tutors with Case Expertise on Problem-Based Learning Issues," *Academic Medicine* 67 (1992):465–469; J. A. Maxwell and L. Wilkerson, "A Study of Non-Volunteer Faculty in a Problem-Based Curriculum," *Academic Medicine* 65(9) (suppl.) (1990):S13–S14.

9. S. P. Mennin and N. Martinez-Burrola, "The Cost of Problem-Based vs. Traditional Medical Education," *Medical Education* 20 (1986):187–194.

10. J. Levinson-Rose and R. J. Menges, "Improving College Teaching: A Critical Review of Research," *Reviews in Educational Research* 51

(1981):403–434; F. T. Stritter, "Faculty Evaluation and Development," in C. McGuire et al., eds., *Handbook of Health Professions Education* (San Francisco: Jossey-Bass, 1983), pp. 294–318.

11. E. H. Schein, *Organizational Culture and Leadership* (San Francisco: Jossey-Bass, 1985).

12. C. R. Christensen, "Premises and Practices of Discussion Teaching," in C. R. Christensen, D. A. Garvin, and A. Sweet, eds., *Education for Judgment: The Artistry of Discussion Leadership* (Boston: Harvard Business School Press, 1991), pp. 15–34.

13. Rogers and Shoemaker, *Communication of Innovations.*

14. A. Kaufman, ed., *Implementing Problem-Based Medical Education: Lessons from Successful Innovations* (New York: Springer-Verlag, 1985).

15. Waugh and Punch, "Teacher Receptivity to Systemwide Change."

16. I. K. Smith, J. O. Smith, and R. P. Durand, "Guidelines for Planning Faculty Development Workshops," *Journal of Biocommunication* 10(2) (1983):8–14.

17. L. Wilkerson, "Identification of Skills for the Problem-Based Tutor: Student and Faculty Perspectives," Paper presented at the annual meeting of the American Educational Research Association, San Francisco, 1992.

18. N. Atebara et al., *The Tutorial Experience: A Survival Guide* (Boston: Harvard Medical School, 1987).

19. Eagle, Harasym, and Mandin, "Effects of Tutors on Problem-Based Learning Issues."

20. L. Wilkerson and J. A. Maxwell, "A Qualitative Study of Initial Faculty Tutors in a Problem-Based Curriculum," *Journal of Medical Education* 63 (1988):892–899.

21. Wilkerson, "Identification of Skills."

22. Wilkerson and Maxwell, "Qualitative Study of Initial Faculty Tutors."

23. L. Wilkerson and J. Boehrer, "Using Cases about Teaching for Faculty Development," in J. Nyquist and D. H. Wulff, eds., *To Improve the Academy: Resources for Student, Faculty, and Institutional Development* (Stillwater, Okla.: New Forums Press, 1992).

24. K. M. Skeff, "Evaluation of a Method for Improving the Teaching Performance of Attending Physicians," *American Journal of Medicine* 75 (1983):465–470; R. J. Menges and K. T. Brinko, "Effects of Student Evaluation Feedback: A Meta-Analysis of Higher Education Research," Paper presented at the annual meeting of the American Educational Research Association, San Francisco, 1986; D. Weinholtz, M. Albanese, R. Zeitler, and G. Everett, "Effects of Individualized Observation with Feedback on Attending Physicians' Clinical Teaching," *Teaching and Learning in Medicine* 1 (1989):128–134.

25. R. M. Harden and F. A. Gleeson, "Assessment of Clinical Competence

Using an Objective Structured Clinical Examination (OSCE)," *Medical Education* 13 (1979):41–54.

26. L. Wilkerson, E. Armstrong, and L. Lesky, "Faculty Development for Ambulatory Teaching," *Journal of General Internal Medicine* 5(1) (suppl.) (1990):S44–S52.

27. A. Bandura, *Social Learning Theory* (Englewood Cliffs, N.J.:Prentice-Hall, 1977).

28. J. Bickel, "The Changing Faces of Promotion and Tenure at U.S. Medical Schools," *Academic Medicine* 66 (1991):249–256.

29. R. M. Rippey, *The Evaluation of Teaching in Medical Schools* (New York: Springer-Verlag, 1981).

8. Project Evaluation

1. M. A. Albanese and S. Mitchell, "Problem-Based Learning: A Review of Literature on Its Outcomes and Implementation Issues," *Academic Medicine* 68 (1993):52–81; D. T. A. Vernon and R. L. Blake, "Does Problem-Based Learning Work? A Meta-Analysis of Evaluative Research," *Academic Medicine* 68 (1993):550–563.

10. Transitional Organization

1. C. R. Christensen, *Teaching and the Case Method* (Boston: Harvard Business School Press, 1987).

13. Lessons for the Future

1. S. Pinker, "Rules of Language," *Science* 253 (1991):530–535.

Contributors

S. James Adelstein, M.D., Ph.D.
Paul C. Cabot Professor of Medical Biophysics
Executive Dean for Academic Programs
Harvard Medical School

Ronald A. Arky, M.D.
Charles C. Davison Professor of Medicine
Master of the Francis Weld Peabody Society, 1987–
Director of Patient–Doctor Sequence, 1988–
Harvard Medical School

Elizabeth G. Armstrong, M.A.T., Ph.D.
Lecturer on Medical Education
Director of Medical Education
Harvard Medical School

G. Octo Barnett, M.D.
Professor of Medicine
Harvard Medical School
Director of Laboratory of Computer Science
Massachusetts General Hospital

Susan D. Block, M.D.
Instructor in Psychiatry
Assistant Director of the New Pathway, 1984–1988
Harvard Medical School

Susan T. Carver, M.D.
Lecturer on Medicine
Special Assistant to Executive Dean for Academic Programs
Harvard Medical School

Henry C. Chueh, M.S., M.D.
Instructor in Medicine
Harvard Medical School
Associate Director of Laboratory of Computer Science
Massachusetts General Hospital

Daniel D. Federman, M.D.
Carl W. Walker Professor of Medicine and Medical Education
Dean for Medical Education
Harvard Medical School

Bruce Forman, M.D.
Research and Clinical Fellow in Medicine
Harvard Medical School
Laboratory of Computer Science
Massachusetts General Hospital

Harvey Goldman, M.D.
Professor of Pathology
Faculty Dean for Medical Education, 1987–1992
Harvard Medical School

Daniel A. Goodenough, Ph.D.
Takeda Professor of Anatomy and Cellular Biology
Master of the Oliver Wendell Holmes Society, 1985–1987, 1992–
Harvard Medical School

Alice S.-H. Huang, Ph.D.
Professor of Microbiology, 1979–1991
Harvard Medical School
Professor of Microbiology and Molecular Genetics
New York University

Robert A. Jenders, M.S., M.D.
Research and Clinical Fellow in Medicine
Harvard Medical School
Laboratory of Computer Science
Massachusetts General Hospital

Patricia J. McArdle, Ed.D., M.S.
Assistant Professor of Social Medicine
Director of Educational Assessment
Coordinator, Patient–Doctor Sequence, 1988–1992
Harvard Medical School

Gordon T. Moore, M.D., M.P.H.
Associate Professor of Ambulatory Care and Prevention
Director of the New Pathway, 1983–1987
Harvard Medical School
Director of Teaching Programs
Harvard Community Health Plan

Judith L. Piggins, M.S.E.E., Ed.M.
Assistant Director of Laboratory of Computer Science
Massachusetts General Hospital

Karla J. Pollick, M.A.
Chief of Staff and Assistant to Dean of the Faculty of Medicine
Associate Director for Planning, 1989–1993
Harvard Medical School

Wayne Raila, B.S.
Lead Programmer of Laboratory of Computer Science
Massachusetts General Hospital

Myra B. Ramos, A.M.
Associate Dean for Educational Services
Assistant to Dean for Academic Programs, 1978–1987
Associate Dean for Educational Planning and Deputy Director of the Office for Educational Development, 1987–1992
Harvard Medical School

Marc T. Silver, M.D.
Research Fellow in Medicine
Student, Oliver Wendell Holmes Society, 1985–1989
Harvard Medical School

August G. Swanson, M.D.
Director of Academic Affairs
Association of American Medical Colleges (through 1991)
Author of *General Professional Education of the Physician,* 1984

Daniel C. Tosteson, M.D.
Caroline Shield Walker Professor of Physiology
Dean of the Faculty of Medicine
Harvard Medical School

LuAnn Wilkerson, Ed.D.
Director of Faculty Development, 1984–1992
Lecturer on Medical Education, 1988–1991
Harvard Medical School
Assistant Dean for Education
Director of Center for Educational Development and Research
University of California, Los Angeles

Index